Clinical Cases in Biochemistry

Clinical Cases in Biochemistry

As per the Revised Competency-based Medical Education Curriculum (NMC-2024)

Second Edition

Ashish Sharma MBBS MD MAMS ACME
Professor and Head
Department of Biochemistry
Geetanjali Medical College and Hospital
Udaipur, Rajasthan, India

Anita Sharma MBBS MD
Professor
Department of Biochemistry
Himalayan Institute of Medical Sciences
Dehradun, Uttarakhand, India

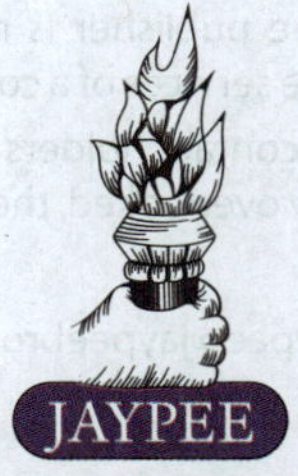

JAYPEE BROTHERS MEDICAL PUBLISHERS
The Health Sciences Publisher
New Delhi | London

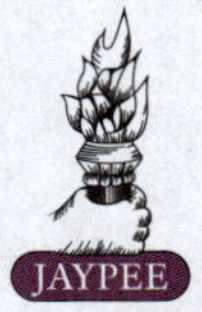

JAYPEE Jaypee Brothers Medical Publishers (P) Ltd.

Headquarters

Jaypee Brothers Medical Publishers (P) Ltd.
EMCA House, 23/23-B
Ansari Road, Daryaganj
New Delhi 110 002, India
Landline: +91-11-23272143, +91-11-23272703
+91-11-23282021, +91-11-23245672
Email: jaypee@jaypeebrothers.com

Corporate Office

Jaypee Brothers Medical Publishers (P) Ltd.
4838/24, Ansari Road, Daryaganj
New Delhi 110 002, India
Phone: +91-11-43574357
Fax: +91-11-43574314
Email: jaypee@jaypeebrothers.com

Overseas Office

J.P. Medical Ltd.
83 Victoria Street, London
SW1H 0HW (UK)
Phone: +44 20 3170 8910
Fax: +44 (0)20 3008 6180
Email: info@jpmedpub.com

Website: www.jaypeebrothers.com
Website: www.jaypeedigital.com

© 2025, Jaypee Brothers Medical Publishers

The views and opinions expressed in this book are solely those of the original contributor(s)/author(s) and do not necessarily represent those of editor(s) and publisher of the book.

All rights reserved. No part of this publication may be reproduced, stored or transmitted in any form or by any means, electronic, mechanical, photocopying, recording or otherwise, without the prior permission in writing of the publishers.

All brand names and product names used in this book are trade names, service marks, trademarks or registered trademarks of their respective owners. The publisher is not associated with any product or vendor mentioned in this book.

Medical knowledge and practice change constantly. This book is designed to provide accurate, authoritative information about the subject matter in question. However, readers are advised to check the most current information available on procedures included and check information from the manufacturer of each product to be administered, to verify the recommended dose, formula, method and duration of administration, adverse effects and contraindications. It is the responsibility of the practitioner to take all appropriate safety precautions. Neither the publisher nor the author(s)/editor(s) assume any liability for any injury and/or damage to persons or property arising from or related to use of material in this book.

This book is sold on the understanding that the publisher is not engaged in providing professional medical services. If such advice or services are required, the services of a competent medical professional should be sought.

Every effort has been made where necessary to contact holders of copyright to obtain permission to reproduce copyright material. If any have been inadvertently overlooked, the publisher will be pleased to make the necessary arrangements at the first opportunity.

Inquiries for bulk sales may be solicited at: jaypee@jaypeebrothers.com

Clinical Cases in Biochemistry

First Edition: 2023

Second Edition: **2025**

ISBN: 978-93-5696-637-6

Printed at Nutech Print Services

Dedicated to

Dr Apurva, Siya and Vasu

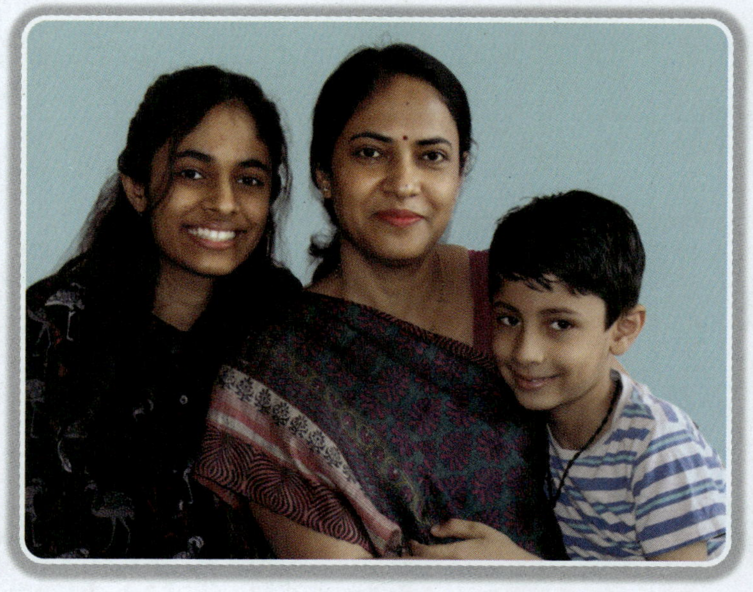

Preface to the Second Edition

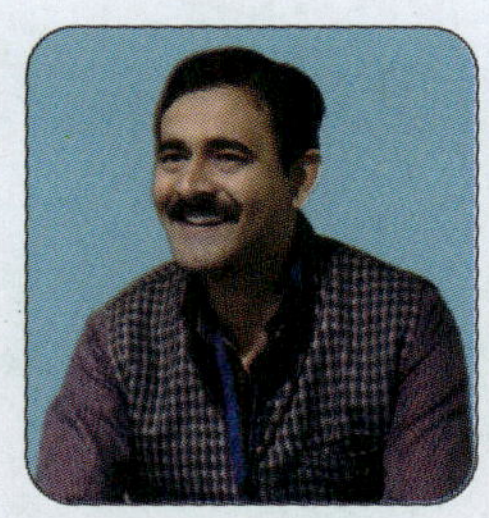

Ashish Sharma

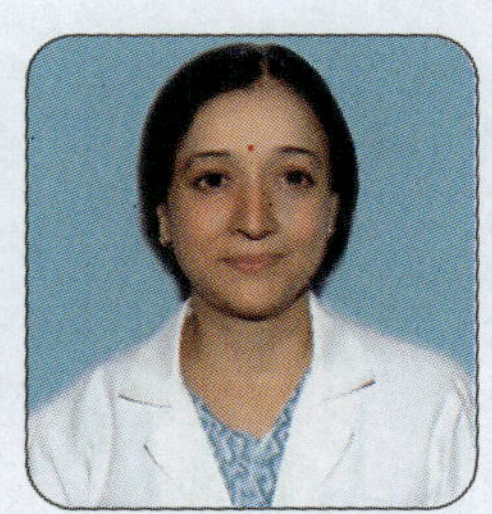

Anita Sharma

To ensure accurate patient management, there is a significant need for a holistic approach that prioritizes teaching and strengthening diagnostic subjects in medical colleges. This is why the National Medical Commission places great emphasis on early clinical exposure, vertical and horizontal integration of teaching subjects, and intermittent formative assessment in competency-based medical education.

With this in mind, we have endeavored to create a straightforward and specialized case-based clinical biochemistry book, enriched with clinical discussions and concise answers aligned with specified competencies. While developing these case studies, we made sure to keep the explanations and narrative clear and simple.

In light of the upcoming NExT pre-PG entrance examination, all case discussions are designed to be concise, focused, and supported by diagrammatic representations of clinical signs and symptoms. We are confident that this book will be valuable to students and aid in clarifying clinical concepts. Feedback and comments are highly appreciated and will be acknowledged in the next edition.

Preface to the First Edition

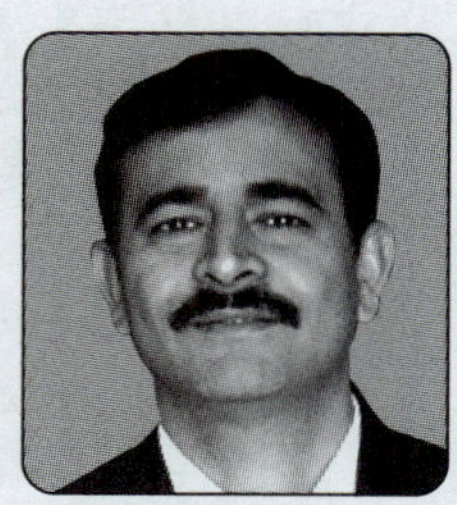

Ashish Sharma

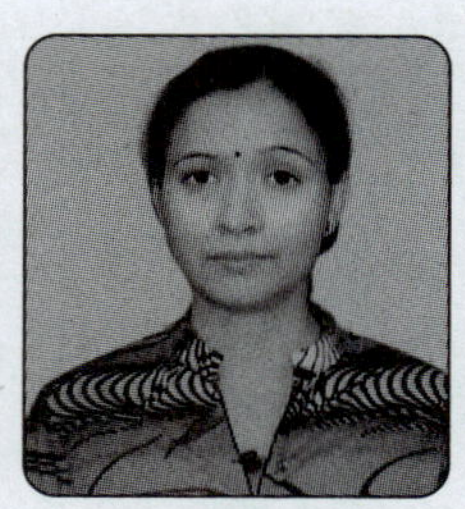

Anita Sharma

For the accurate management of patients, there is a great need of holistic approach, which emphasises teaching and strengthening of diagnostic subjects in medical colleges. That is why, National Medical Commission greatly emphasis on early clinical exposure, vertical and horizontal integration of teaching subjects, intermittent formative assessment in competency based medical education.

In this context, we made an effort to provide a simple and exclusive case based clinical biochemistry book enriched with clinical discussion, short answers with the specified competencies.

While developing case studies in clinical biochemistry, special precaution has been taken to keep the explanation and narration simple.

In the light of upcoming NExT pre-PG entrance examination, all the case discussions are crisp, to the point with diagrammatic representation of clinical signs and symptoms.

We are confident that this book will be useful for all the students and helpful in making their clinical concepts clear. Feedback and comments are most welcomed and will be duly acknowledged in the next edition.

Acknowledgments

We are delighted to announce the second edition of *Clinical Cases in Biochemistry*! Writing this book has been a journey of learning and discovery, and we are indebted to many people who have supported me along the way.

We are deeply grateful to **Almighty God**; whose divine guidance illuminate every step of this journey.

*To my **Parents** for their love, care and support.*

*To my wife **Dr Apurva**, who has been my pillar of strength, her insights and feedback have shaped this work in more ways than I can express.*

*To my sister and co-author **Dr Anita**, whose guidance and expertize has been invaluable throughout this process.*

*To my kids **Siya and Vasu** for their unwavering support and love through my tough times.*

*I am also profoundly thankful to my colleagues **Dr Sohil, Dr Jaswanth, Dr Rishab, Vinay, Deepti, Pooja, Naval and my students Manish, Ravinandan, Meghna, Khwaish,** those provided steady support and for their patience during the long hours and challenging moments. Their belief in me has been my anchor.*

Ashish Sharma

I extend my heartfelt gratitude to my parents, teachers, colleagues, and students for their constant support and blessings.

*A special thanks to **Dr Vijay Dhasmana**, our esteemed President of SRHU University, **Dr Rajendra Dobhal**, Vice-President and **Dr Vijendra D Chauhan**, Director-Genera of Academics, for their invaluable guidance and support. Your mentorship has been instrumental in shaping my research and writing journey.*

*I also want to express my deepest appreciation to **Prof (Dr) AK Deorari**, our esteemed Principal, for fostering an environment of academic excellence and providing valuable insights for this publication.*

*Lastly, I extend my sincere thanks to **Dr Rajesh Agarwal**, a renowned pediatrician in Rishikesh, for taking the time to review the book and offer his invaluable suggestions.*

Anita Sharma

We are also very grateful to the whole team of M/s Jaypee Brothers Medical Publishers (P) Ltd, New Delhi, India, who helped and guided me, Shri Jitendar P Vij (Group Chairman), Mr Ankit Vij (Managing Director), Mr MS Mani (Group President), Dr Madhu Choudhary (Director–Educational Publishing), Ms Pooja Bhandari [Director–Production (Books and Journals)], Mr Ajay Kumar Sharma [Deputy General Manager (Books and Journals)], Ms Sunita Katla (Executive Assistant to Group Chairman and Publishing Manager),

Ms Samina Khan (Executive Assistant to Director–Educational Publishing), Dr Aditya Tayal (Editorial Manager–Content Strategy), Ms Seema Dogra (Cover Visualizer), Ms Neha Verma (Graphic Designer–Cover), Ms Neelam Kakriya (Proofreader), Mr Manoj Pahuja (Graphic Designer) and Mr Kuldeep Dobriyal (Typesetter) , for all their support to work in this project and make it a success. Without their cooperation, I could not have completed this project.

Lastly, we want to thank our students. This book exists because of their curiosity, passion, and willingness to explore new ideas. We hope it serves as a source of inspiration and insight.

Thank you all for your unwavering support and encouragement. This book stands as a testament to our collective efforts and dedication to the pursuit of knowledge.

Contents

Section 1: Carbohydrate Metabolism

Section 2: Protein Metabolism

Section 3: Lipid Metabolism

Section 4: Vitamins

Section 5: Minerals

Section 6: Enzymes

Section 7: Heme and Hemoglobin Metabolism

Section 8: Hormones

Section 9: Water, Electrolyte, and Acid Base Balance

Section 10: Nucleic Acid Metabolism

Section 11: Miscellaneous

Competency Table

Competency number	*Competency*	*Case number*	*Page number*
BC2.3	Describe enzyme inhibition and the role of enzymes or drugs as inhibitors and therapeutic agents	6.2, 6.5	148, 155
BC2.4	Describe and discuss the clinical utility of various serum enzymes in laboratory and their use as markers of pathological conditions	6.1, 6.4	143, 153
BC2.5	Interpret laboratory results of enzymes in various disorders	6.1	143
BC3.2	Describe the digestion, absorption, and transport of carbohydrates from food along with associated disorders	1.6	22
BC3.3	Define and briefly describe the pathways of carbohydrate metabolism and their regulation (glycolysis, gluconeogenesis, TCA, and significance of glycogen metabolism and HMP shunt), with associated disorders	1.3	11
BC3.4	Describe regulation, functions, and integration of carbohydrate metabolism, including disorders	1.3	11
BC3.5	Discuss the mechanism and significance of blood glucose regulation in health and disease	1.2, 1.4, 1.5	7, 15, 19
BC3.6	Interpret the results of analytes associated with carbohydrate metabolism and laboratory investigations related to carbohydrate disorders	1.1, 1.2	3, 7
BC4.1	Describe and discuss main classes of lipids and their functions	3.5, 3.7	75, 79
BC4.2	Describe digestion and absorption of dietary lipids and associated disorders	3.1	63
BC4.4	Describe triglyceride and cholesterol metabolism and clinical significance	3.1, 3.3	63, 70
BC4.5	Describe the metabolism of lipoproteins with brief overview of lipoprotein structure, their interrelations & relations with atherosclerosis	6.1	143
BC4.6	Discuss biological role and therapeutic applications of Eicosanoids and their Inhibitors	3.5	75
BC4.7	Describe fatty liver, cholelithiasis, and obesity	3.2	66
BC4.8	Interpret laboratory results of analytes associated with metabolism of Lipids	3.2, 3.4, 3.6, 3.8	66, 73, 77, 82
BC5.4	Describe plasma proteins and their functions, including electrophoretic patterns and acute phase proteins	2.4	45

Competency number	*Competency*	*Case number*	*Page number*
BC5.6	Describe the formation, transport, detoxification of Ammonia, Ammonia toxicity and its clinical significance	2.7	54
BC5.7	Describe the specialized products formed from the amino acids Glycine, Phenylalanine, Tyrosine, Tryptophan, and Methionine, branched chain amino acids and Arginine and the inborn errors associated with them. Discuss newborn screening	2.1, 2.2, 2.3, 2.5	35, 38, 42, 48
BC5.8	Describe the structure and functions of haem and its metabolism, with emphasis on jaundice and porphyrin metabolism	7.1, 7.2	163, 167
BC5.9	Describe major types of hemoglobin, their derivatives, and physiological/pathological relevance	7.6, 7.7	178, 180
BC6.1	Enumerate the functions and components of the extracellular matrix (ECM)	1.7	26
BC6.2	Discuss the involvement of ECM components in health and disease	1.7	26
BC8.1	Describe biochemical role of vitamins and manifestations of their deficiency	4.1, 4.2, 4.3, 4.4, 4.5, 4.6, 4.7, 4.8, 4.9	89, 92, 95, 98, 101, 105, 109, 112, 115
BC8.3	Describe the types and causes of protein-energy malnutrition and its effects	2.6	51
BC8.5	Describe causes, effects, and health risks associated with overweight, obesity, and metabolic syndrome	8.3	194
BC9.1	Describe the dietary sources, absorption, transport, and metabolism of iron, calcium, and copper, including their clinical disorders	5.1, 5.2, 5.3	125, 128, 131
BC9.2	Discuss magnesium, zinc, and phosphorus, their clinical significance, and functions of trace elements	5.4, 5.5	134, 137
BC9.3	Describe processes involved in maintaining normal pH, water, and electrolyte balance, and derangements associated with them	1.2, 9.1, 9.2, 9.3, 9.4, 9.5	7, 201, 203, 205, 208, 211
BC10.1	Describe nucleotides and nucleic acids and their clinical significance	10.3	224
BC10.2	Describe briefly the synthesis of purines with special emphasis on the salvage pathway	10.1, 10.2	217, 222
BC10.3	Describe degradation of purines and its significance, including associated disorders	10.1, 10.2	217, 222
BC11.1	Describe function tests of kidney, liver, thyroid, and adrenal glands, and interpret their function tests	8.1, 8.2, 11.2	189, 192, 238
BC11.2	Enumerate the hormones and markers related to reproduction and reproductive health and their clinical interpretation (e.g., LH, FSH, prolactin, beta-HCG, estrogen, progesterone, testosterone and AMH). Discuss importance of prenatal screening	8.3	194

Competency number	Competency	Case number	Page number
BC12.3	Describe the role of oxidative stress in the pathogenesis of conditions such as cancer, complications of diabetes mellitus and atherosclerosis	6.1	143
BC13.4	Discuss metabolism of alcohol with biochemical changes and effects of chronic alcoholism	3.2	66
BC14.2	Describe estimation of pH-by-pH meter or ABG analyzer and interpret results with paper case scenarios	1.2, 9.2, 9.3, 9.4, 9.5	7, 203, 205, 208, 211
BC14.17	Briefly describe various body fluids and discuss the composition of cerebrospinal fluid (CSF)	11.1	235
BC14.19	Explain the basis and rationale of biochemical tests done and interpretation of results in various conditions	2.4, 3.3, 5.4, 6.3, 7.3, 7.4, 7.5, 8.1, 8.2, 11.2, 11.3	45, 70, 134, 151, 169, 172, 175, 189, 192, 238, 241
Integration with Pathology			
PA16.2	Describe the pathogenesis, features, hematologic indices, and peripheral blood picture of sickle cell anemia and thalassemia	7.6, 7.7	178, 180
PA24.1	Describe bilirubin metabolism and pathogenesis of jaundice, distinguishing between direct and indirect hyperbilirubinemia	7.3, 7.4, 7.5	169, 172, 175
Integration with Medicine			
GM2.1	Discuss and describe the epidemiology, antecedents, and risk factors for atherosclerosis and ischemic heart disease	6.1	143
GM2.3	Discuss and describe the lipid cycle and the role of dyslipidemia in the pathogenesis of atherosclerosis	6.1	143
GM4.6	Discuss the approach to the patient with Acute Febrile Illness	11.1	235
GM5.1	Describe and discuss the physiologic and biochemical basis of hyperbilirubinemia	7.3, 7.4, 7.5	169, 172, 175
GM5.3	Describe and discuss the epidemiology, microbiology, immunology, and clinical evolution of infective (viral) hepatitis	6.4	153
GM5.5	Describe and discuss the pathophysiology, clinical evolution, and complications of cirrhosis and portal hypertension	2.7	54
GM5.6	Enumerate and describe the causes and pathophysiology of drug induced liver injury	6.2	148
GM7.3	Develop a systematic clinical approach to joint pain based on the pathophysiology	10.1	217
GM9.2	Describe the morphological characteristics, etiology, and prevalence of anemia	1.3	11

Competency number	*Competency*	*Case number*	*Page number*
GM9.9	Describe and develop a diagnostic plan to determine the etiology of anemia	5.2	128
GM9.16	Communicate and counsel patients on methods to prevent nutritional anemia	5.2	128
GM10.1	Define, describe, classify, differentiate between the pathophysiologic causes of acute and chronic renal failure	11.3	241
GM10.5	Describe the pathophysiology and clinical findings of uraemia	11.2	238
GM11.5	Describe and discuss the pathogenesis and temporal evolution of microvascular and macrovascular complications of diabetes	1.1	3
GM11.9	Describe and recognize the clinical features of patients who present with a diabetic emergency	1.2	7
GM12.1	Describe the epidemiology, genetic basis and pathogenesis of hypothyroidism and hyperthyroidism including the influence of iodine deficiency and autoimmunity in the pathogenesis of thyroid disease	8.1, 8.2	189, 192
GM13.14	Describe the indications for surgery, radiation and chemotherapy for common malignancies	10.3	224
GM16.2	Describe and discuss the acute systemic consequences of diarrhea including its impact on fluid balance	9.1	201
GM17.7	Enumerate the indication of lumbar puncture and describe the findings in CSF in different types of meningitis	11.1	235
GM22.4	Enumerate and describe commonly observed drug overdoses, toxicology, clinical features, prognosis, and therapy	6.5	155
GM23.4	Enumerate causes, describe clinical features, and provide correct diagnosis and management approach for hyponatremia	1.2	7
GM23.8	Enumerate causes and describe clinical and laboratory features of metabolic acidosis	1.2, 9.4	7, 208
GM23.9	Enumerate the causes and describe the clinical and laboratory features of metabolic alkalosis	9.5	211
GM23.10	Enumerate the causes and describe the clinical and laboratory features of respiratory acidosis	9.2	203
GM23.11	Enumerate the causes and describe the clinical and laboratory features of respiratory alkalosis	9.3	205
GM24.3	Discuss and describe the etiology, causes, clinical manifestations, complications, diagnosis, and management of common vitamin deficiencies	4.1, 4.2, 4.3, 4.4, 4.5, 4.6, 4.7, 4.8, 4.9	89, 92, 95, 98, 101, 105, 109, 112, 115

Competency number	*Competency*	*Case number*	*Page number*
GM26.12	Describe and discuss the common causes, clinical features and management of encephalitis and meningitis	11.1	235
Integration with Pediatrics			
PE10.2	Outline the clinical approach to a child with SAM and MAM	2.6	51
PE10.3	Assessment of a patient with SAM and MAM, including classification, diagnosis, and management	2.6	51
PE12.1	Discuss RDA, dietary sources, and role of vitamin A in health and disease	4.7	109
PE12.2	Describe causes, clinical features, diagnosis, and management of deficiency/excess of vitamin A	4.7	109
PE12.3	Describe causes, clinical features, diagnosis, and management of deficiency/excess of vitamin D (Rickets and Hypervitaminosis D)	4.8	112
PE12.5	Describe the RDA, dietary sources of Vitamin K and their role in health and disease	4.9	115
PE12.6	Describe the causes, clinical features, diagnosis, management and prevention of deficiency of Vitamin K	4.9	115
PE12.7	Describe causes, clinical features, diagnosis, and management of deficiency of B complex vitamins	4.1, 4.2, 4.3, 4.4, 4.5	89, 92, 95, 98, 101
PE12.8	Describe RDA, dietary sources, and management of vitamin C deficiency	4.6	105
PE13.3	Describe the RDA, dietary sources of Iodine and their role in Health and disease, deficiency, and Goiter control program	5.4	134
PE13.4	Describe the RDA, dietary sources, and role of calcium and magnesium in health and deficiency states	5.1	125
PE19.5	Describe etiology, clinical features, and management of respiratory distress in newborns	3.7	79
PE19.15	Describe the etiology, clinical features, and management of neonatal hyperbilirubinemia	1.3, 1.4	11, 15
PE23.4	Define diarrhea (acute diarrhea, chronic diarrhea, persistent diarrhea). Discuss etiology, risk factors, clinical features, complications, investigations and treatment (according to WHO guidelines) of acute gastroenteritis	1.6	22

Section 1

Carbohydrate Metabolism

Case 1.1

Diabetes Mellitus

COMPETENCY

❖ **BC3.6:** Interpret the results of analytes associated with metabolism of carbohydrates and other laboratory investigations related to disorders of carbohydrate metabolism

Integration with Medicine

❖ **GM11.5:** Describe and discuss the pathogenesis and temporal evolution of microvascular and macrovascular complications of diabetes

Case Scenario

A middle-aged individual complains of excessive thirst (polydipsia), excessive hunger (polyphagia) and excessive urination (polyuria) **(Fig. 1.1.1)**.

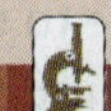

Laboratory Findings Reveal

- Random blood sugar: 180 mg/dL
- Urine is positive for sugar in dipstick test

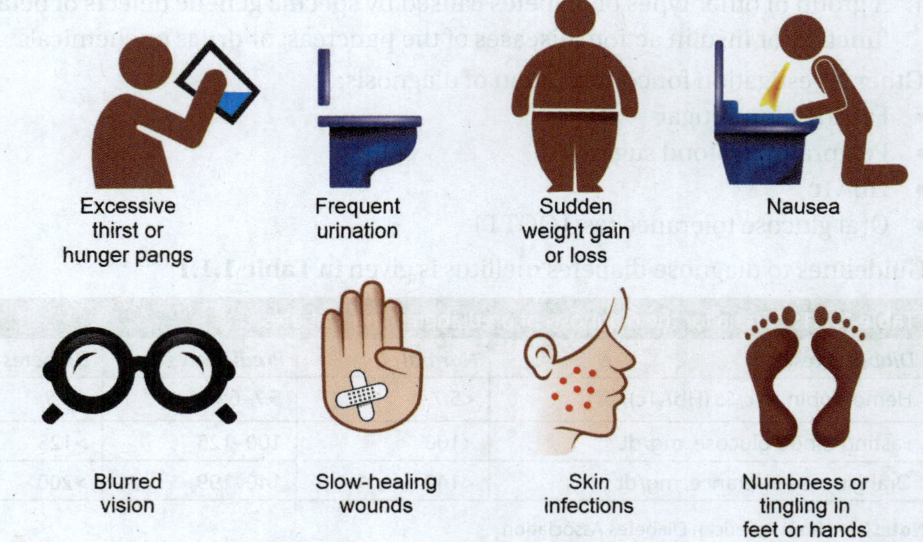

Fig. 1.1.1: Clinical presentation of diabetes mellitus.

QUESTIONS

Q.1. What is your diagnosis, what other investigations you would like to add to confirm your diagnosis?

Q.2. What is the guideline for diagnosis of diabetes mellitus?

Q.3. Explain the biochemical basis of the clinical symptoms.

Q.4. Which is the investigation of choice for the diagnosis and follow up of diabetic patients and why?

Q.5. What are the complications in uncontrolled diabetes mellitus? What is the management for diabetic patients?

ANSWERS

A.1. This patient is probably suffering with diabetes mellitus.

Diabetes mellitus is a group of chronic metabolic conditions, all of which are characterized by elevated blood glucose levels resulting from the body's inability to produce insulin or resistance to insulin action, or both. This group of conditions can be subdivided into four clinically distinct types:

1. Type 1, which results from autoimmune beta-cell destruction in the pancreas and is characterized by a complete lack of insulin production
2. Type 2, which develops when there is an abnormal increased resistance to the action of insulin and the body cannot produce enough insulin to overcome the resistance
3. Gestational diabetes, which is a form of glucose intolerance that affects some women during pregnancy
4. A group of other types of diabetes caused by specific genetic defects of beta-cell function or insulin action, diseases of the pancreas, or drugs or chemicals

Other investigation for confirmation of diagnosis:

- Fasting blood sugar
- Postprandial blood sugar
- HbA1c
- Oral glucose tolerance test (OGTT)

A.2. Guidelines to diagnose diabetes mellitus is given in **Table 1.1.1**

Table 1.1.1: Criteria for the diagnosis of prediabetes and diabetes.

Diabetes test	*Normal*	*Prediabetes*	*Diabetes*
Hemoglobin A1c, % (HbA1c)	<5.7	5.7–6.4	>6.5
Fasting blood glucose, mg/dL	<100	100–125	>125
Oral glucose tolerance, mg/dL	<140	140–199	>200

Note: Data from American Diabetes Association.

(A1c-glycated hemoglobin)

A.3. Explain the biochemical basis of the clinical symptoms.

Polyphagia (excessive eating): Due to lack of insulin cells are deprived of glucose and also fails to produce adequate ATP, thus patient constantly feels hungry and eats too much.

Polyuria (excessive urination): Hyperglycemia (high levels of blood glucose) when reaches above renal threshold, it comes out in urine and glucose concentration increases in lumen. Glucose is osmotically active cause drawing of water from renal epithelial cells, causes increase volume of urine (polyuria), which further due to depletion of water in body results in **polydipsia**.

A.4. For a naive case confirmatory diagnostic test is oral glucose tolerance test (OGTT) and for a known case of diabetes, glycated hemoglobin (HbA1c) is the investigation of choice for follow up of patients.

A.5. Diabetes leads to micro and macrovascular complications in long uncontrolled cases **(Fig. 1.1.2)**.

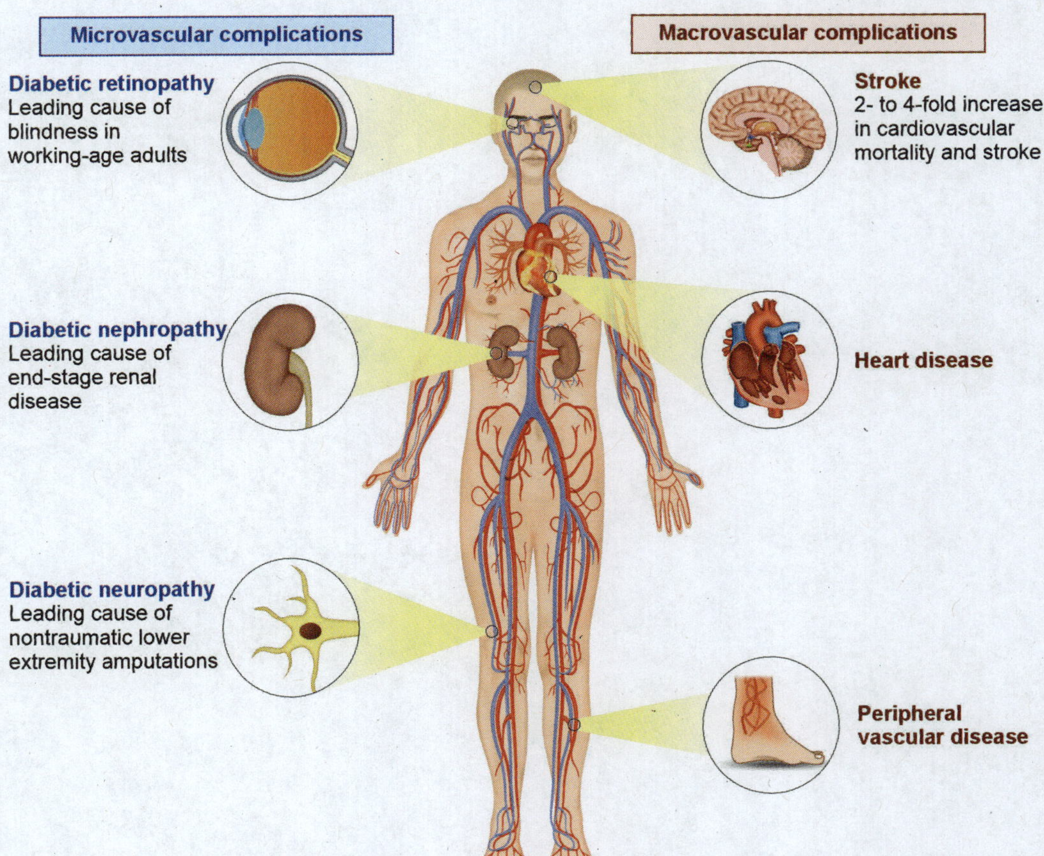

Fig. 1.1.2: Complications of diabetes.

Management of Diabetes Patients

Diabetic patients must take responsibility for their day-to-day care. This includes monitoring blood glucose levels, dietary management, maintaining physical activity, keeping weight and stress under control, monitoring oral medications and if required, insulin use via injections or pump.

BIBLIOGRAPHY

1. American Diabetes Association. Diagnosis and classification of diabetes mellitus. Diabetes Care. 2010;33 (Suppl 1):S62-9.
2. Deshpande AD, Harris-Hayes M, Schootman M. Epidemiology of diabetes and diabetes-related complications. Phys Ther. 2008;88(11):1254-64.
3. National Center for Health Statistics, Centers for Disease Control and Prevention. National Health Interview Survey. Available at: http://www.cdc.gov/nchs/nhis.htm

Case 1.2

Diabetic Ketoacidosis

COMPETENCY

- **BC3.5:** Discuss the mechanism and significance of blood glucose regulation (glucose homeostasis) in health and disease. Describe the types, biochemical changes, complications and laboratory investigations related to diabetes and other carbohydrate metal disorders
- **BC3.6:** Interpret the results of analytes associated with metabolism of carbohydrates and other laboratory investigations related to disorders of carbohydrate metabolism
- **BC9.3:** Describe the processes involved in maintenance of normal pH, water and electrolyte balance of body fluids and the derangements associated with them
- **BC14.2:** Describe estimation of pH-by-pH meter or ABG analyser and interpretation of results with paper case scenarios

Integration with Medicine

- **GM11.9:** Describe and recognise the clinical features of patients who present with a diabetic emergency
- **GM23.4:** Enumerate the causes and describe the clinical features and the correct approach to the diagnosis and management for a patient with hyponatremia
- **GM23.8:** Enumerate the causes and describe the clinical and laboratory features of metabolic acidosis

Case Scenario

A 5-year-old girl was brought to hospital in unconscious state. Her mother stated that the girl was apparently well about 2 weeks back when she developed a sore throat and mild fever and started to feel generally unwell. The child was treated by pediatrician. Several days before admission, she began to complain of undue thirst and also started to get up several times at night to urinate. However on the day of admission she had abdominal pain, started to vomit, her breathing was rapid and deep, and become drowsy.

On examination, she was dehydrated, skin was cold, had deep sighing breathing. Breath had fruity odor, heart rate 120/min, BP-90/60.

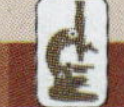

Laboratory Findings Reveal

- Plasma glucose : 520 mg/dL (70–140 mg/dL)
- Arterial blood pH : 7.02 (7.35–7.45)
- Na^+ : 130 mmol/L (136–145 mmol/L)
- K^+ : 5.9 mmol/L (3.5–5.0 mmol/L)
- Cl^- : 100 mmol/L (96–106 mmol/L)

Urinalysis

- Glucose : ++++
- Keto acids : ++++

QUESTIONS

Q.1. What is the most probable diagnosis? Explain how you reach on your diagnosis. What could be the precipitating cause of this condition?

Q.2. Patient present with which type of homeostatic imbalance (acid-base imbalance) and enumerate four other important clinical conditions that leads to same metabolic dysfunction.

Q.3. Explain, why patient experienced a typical rapid and deep (hyperventilated) breathing.

Q.4. Which electrolyte needs to be closely monitored and why?

Q.5. Why there is excess formation of ketone bodies in diabetic ketoacidosis?

Q.6. Name the tests done to detect ketone bodies in urine.

ANSWERS

A.1. Child is suffering from Type 1 diabetes mellitus with diabetic ketoacidosis. Diabetic ketoacidosis (DKA) is a serious complication of diabetes that can be life-threatening. DKA is most common among people with Type 1 diabetes.

Child with typical laboratory finding of hyperglycemia, presence of urinary glucose and ketone with typical history, presenting complains and symptoms **(Fig. 1.2.1)** confirms the diagnosis of Type-1 diabetes (juvenile) mellitus with ketoacidosis.

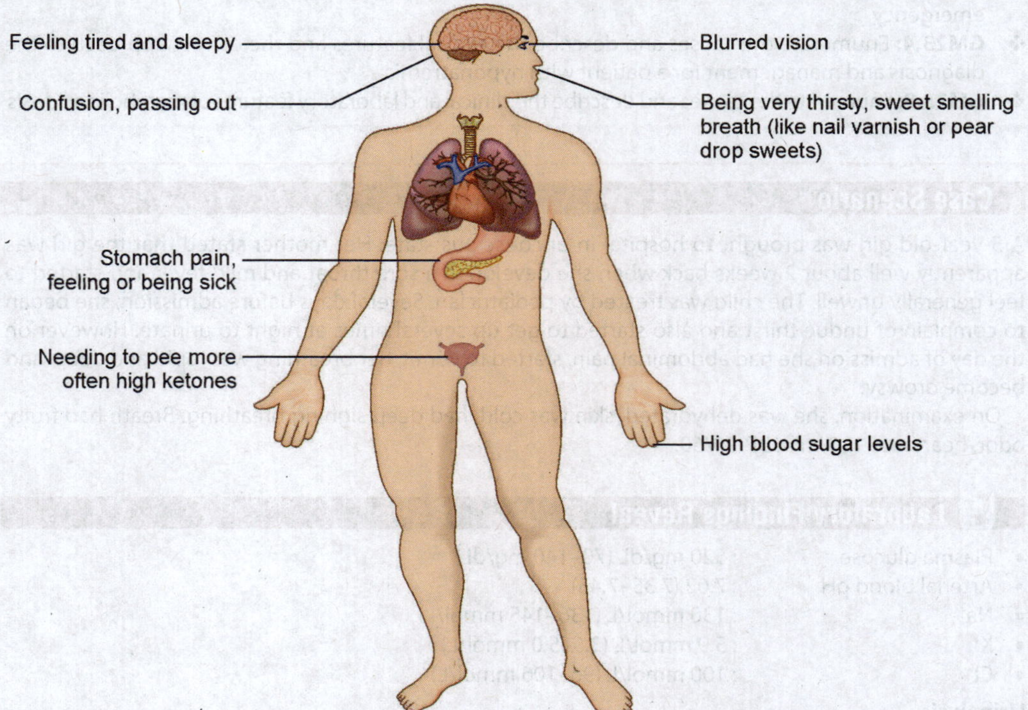

Fig. 1.2.1: Presenting complains, signs and symptoms of patients with diabetic ketoacidosis.

Precipitating cause can be acute viral infection. Autoimmunity to β-cell is initiated by a viral protein can have etiological role in disease development. Other precipitating factors—genetic susceptibility and other host factors like HLA-DR3 or DR-4.

A.2. Patient is suffering from metabolic acidosis (diabetic ketoacidosis) due to excessive formation of ketone bodies. Ketone bodies are acid in nature.

Other causes of ketoacidosis:

- Starvation
- Toxemia of pregnancy
- Physical or emotional trauma
- Heart attack or stroke
- Pancreatitis
- Alcohol and drug abuse particularly cocaine
- Inadequate insulin dose
- Medications like corticosteroids

A.3. Typical breathing pattern in diabetic ketoacidosis is k/a "Kussmaul breathing" which is a compensatory mechanism to restore homeostasis characterized by hyperventilation. Hyperventilation occurs to remove CO_2 from the body and reduces the acid load (H_2CO_3). In an attempt to expel carbon dioxide, which is an acidic compound in blood, the body starts to breathe faster and deeper. Kussmaul breathing is **characterized by a deep, rapid breathing pattern**. It is typically an indication that the body or organs have become too acidic.

A.4. Insulin promotes potassium entry into cells. When circulating insulin is lacking, as in DKA, potassium moves out of cells, thus raising plasma potassium levels even in the presence of total body potassium deficiency. After insulin treatment is initiated, potassium shifts intracellularly and serum levels decline, replacement of potassium in intravenous fluids is the standard of care in treatment of DKA to prevent the potential consequences of hypokalemia including cardiac arrhythmias and respiratory failure.

A.5. The combination of hyperglycemia, glycosuria, ketonuria and ketonemia is called diabetic ketoacidosis. Even though glucose is in excess, not available to the extrahepatic cell due to the deficiency of insulin. It may further accelerates lipolysis in extrahepatic tissues, increases free fatty acid in the circulation. Oxidation of fatty acids increases acetyl-CoA pool. Enhanced gluconeogenesis in the liver causes limited availability of oxaloacetate and restricts the oxidation of acetyl-CoA. Accumulated acetyl-CoA diverts towards ketone body formation.

A.6. Most urinalysis reagent tests utilize the nitroprusside test (Rothera's test).

Which is most sensitive to acetoacetate, less sensitive to acetone and not sensitive to beta-hydroxybutyric acid

False positive Rothera's test: Heavily pigmented urine. Drugs such as captopril, L-dopa, salicylates, phenothiazines.

False negative Rothera's test: Negative nitroprusside tests for ketonuria underestimate the presence of ketonemia due to increased beta-hydroxybutyric acid concentrations.

BIBLIOGRAPHY

1. American Diabetes Association. Diagnosis and classification of diabetes mellitus. Diabetes Care. 2006;29:S43–S48.
2. https://www.cdc.gov/diabetes/basics/diabetic-ketoacidosis.html

Case 1.3

G6PD Deficiency

COMPETENCY

- ❖ **BC3.3:** Define and briefly describe the pathways of carbohydrate metabolism and their regulation (glycolysis, gluconeogenesis, TCA, and significance of glycogen metabolism and HMP shunt), with associated disorders
- ❖ **BC3.4:** Describe and discuss the regulation, functions and integration of minor carbohydrate metabolism pathway briefly along with associated diseases/disorders

Integration with Medicine

- ❖ **GM9.2:** Describe and discuss the morphological characteristics, etiology and prevalence of each of the causes of anemia

Integration with Pediatrics

- ❖ **PE19.15:** Describe the etiology, clinical features and management of neonatal hyperbilirubinemia

Case Scenario

A 20-year-old male suffering from malaria was treated with primaquine and presents with history of sudden onset of fatigue, breathlessness, pale skin, abdominal discomfort, laboratory finding reveals **(Fig. 1.3.1)**.

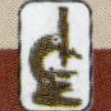

Laboratory Findings Reveal

Test	*Results*	*Normal range*
Hemoglobin	8 g%	12–16 g%
Total bilirubin	4.8 mg/dL	0.2–1.2 mg/dL
Indirect bilirubin	4.0 mg/dL	0.2–0.7 mg/dL
SGOT	126 IU/L	8–20 IU/L
SGPT	78 IU/L	10–40 IU/L

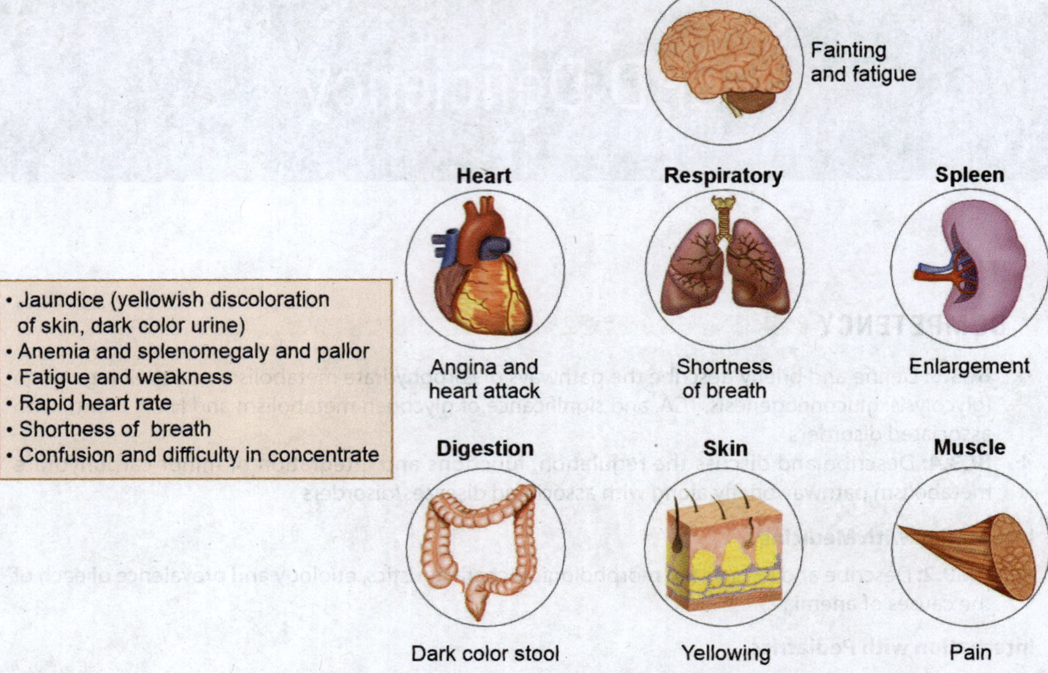

Fig. 1.3.1: Clinical presentation of G6PD deficiency.

QUESTIONS

Q.1. What is the most probable diagnosis of the patient? Explain biochemical basis of this clinical presentation.

Q.2. What is the confirmatory diagnosis?

Q.3. What is favism?

Q.4. Enumerate other factors which may precipitate acute hemolytic anemia in these patients.

ANSWERS

A.1. This patient is suffering from hemolytic anemia with jaundice due to glucose-6 phosphate dehydrogenase enzyme deficiency. G6PD deficiency is a genetic disorder with X-linked recessive inheritance.

G6PD is the rate regulating enzyme of HMP shunt pathway, which provides two important biomolecules reducing bioequivalent NADPH + H, pentose sugar.

G6PD deficient patient has compromised NADPH levels which is essential in maintenance of RBC membrane integrity by maintaining reduced glutathione levels, protection from free radical injury **(Fig. 1.3.2A)**.

Table 1.3.1: Physiological importance of HMP shunt.
◆ To produce NADPH which is required for: - Reductive biosynthesis—fatty acids, cholesterol and steroid hormones - Free radical scavenging - Maintain RBC membrane integrity by keeping GSH in reduced state - Prevention of methemoglobin formation - Detoxification by hydroxylation - Maintain the transparency of lens - Bactericidal activity of macrophages ◆ To produce ribose and deoxyribose for DNA and RNA synthesis

Drugs like antimalarials has precipitated oxidative stress resulting in an attack of hemolytic anemia and breathlessness, pale skin followed by jaundice.

A.2. Blood G6PD enzyme levels are the confirmatory test. Other diagnostic tests that may be done include atypical peripheral blood smear specially blister cells, bite cells **(Fig. 1.3.2B)**, complete blood count, serum hemoglobin test, and a reticulocyte count.

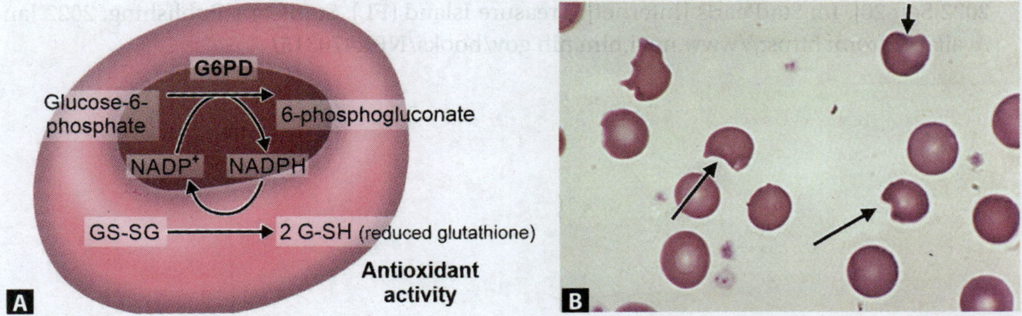

Figs. 1.3.2A and B: (A) Generation of reduced form of glutathione; (B) Peripheral blood film in G6PD deficiency.

A.3. Ingestion of toxic glycosides present in fava beans stimulates peroxides formation inside RBC. In G6PD deficient cells the level of NADPH is low; hence further production of peroxides will lead to cell lysis **(Figs. 1.3.3A and B)**.

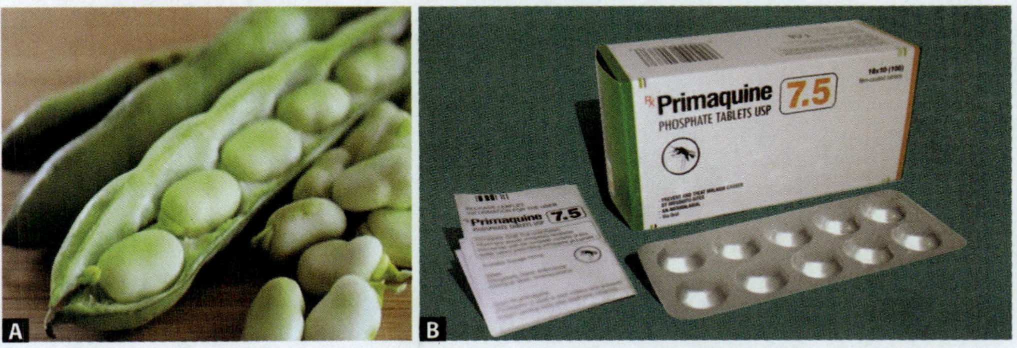

Figs. 1.3.3A and B: Factor which precipitate symptoms of G6PD deficiency: (A) Fava bean; (B) Antimalarial drug, primaquine.

A.4. Factor which precipitate symptoms of G6PD deficiency are:
- Antimalarials, sulfonamide, aspirin
- Nonsteroidal anti-inflammatory medications (NSAIDs)
- Eating fava beans or certain legumes.

People which may at higher risk of having G6PD deficiency:
- Male
- African-American
- Middle Eastern descent
- Family history of the condition

BIBLIOGRAPHY

1. Avalos S, Mejia RE, Banegas E, Salinas C, Gutierrez L, Fajardo M, Galo S, Pinto A, Mejia A, Fontecha G. G6PD deficiency, primaquine treatment, and risk of haemolysis in malaria-infected patients. Malar J. 2018;17(1):415.
2. Richardson SR, O'Malley GF. Glucose-6-Phosphate Dehydrogenase Deficiency. [Updated 2022 Sep 26]. In: StatPearls [Internet]. Treasure Island (FL): StatPearls Publishing; 2022 Jan-. Available from: https://www.ncbi.nlm.nih.gov/books/NBK470315/

Case 1.4

Galactosemia

COMPETENCY

- **BC3.5:** Discuss the mechanism and significance of blood glucose regulation (glucose homeostasis) in health and disease. Describe the types, biochemical changes, complications and laboratory investigations related to diabetes and other carbohydrate metal disorders

Integration with Pediatrics

- **PE19.15:** Describe the etiology, clinical features and management of neonatal hyperbilirubinemia

Case Scenario

A male infant weighing 3.1 kilograms was delivered at 38 weeks to a 34-year-old woman, gravida 3, para 1. He was discharged home in good health 24 hours post-delivery. However, two days later, he presented at the outpatient clinic with jaundice. On examination, no hepatosplenomegaly was noted. His indirect bilirubin level was 23.1 mg/dL, and his blood group was Rh positive. An exchange blood transfusion was performed, and he was discharged after two days **(Fig. 1.4.1)**.

The baby was readmitted to the NICU with complaints of fever (38.5°C), vomiting, dehydration, and jaundice. Physical examination revealed decreased muscle tone, jaundice, and hepatomegaly. Laboratory findings showed blood glucose levels of 60 mg/dL, total bilirubin of 15 mg/dL, blood urea of 150 mg/dL, and serum uric acid of 9.0 mg/dL. Blood culture revealed *E. coli* growth.

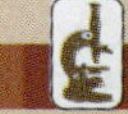

Laboratory Findings Reveal

Biochemical investigations show:

- Blood glucose—60 mg/dL (70–140 mg/dL)
- Total bilirubin—2.00 mg/dL (0.2–1.2 mg/dL)
- Serum uric acid—8.1 mg/dL (3.5–7.2 mg/dL)
- Reducing sugar present in urine

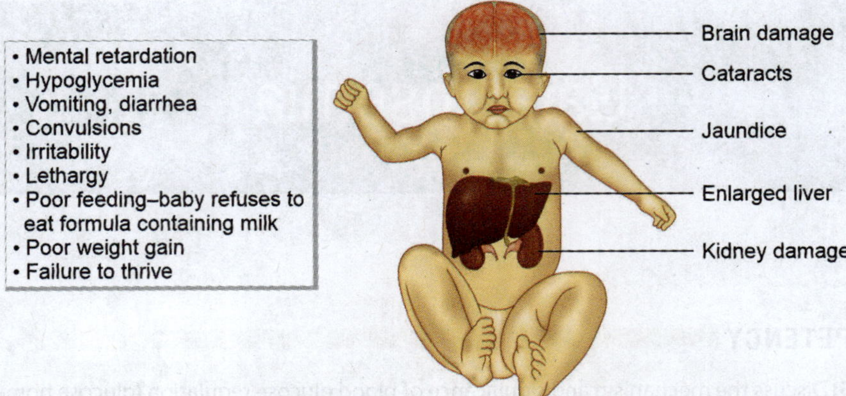

Fig.1.4.1: Clinical presentation of galactosemia.

QUESTIONS

Q.1. What is the probable diagnosis? Explain metabolic defects in such clinical condition.

Q.2. Explain biochemical basis of signs and symptoms of this condition.

Q.3. Enumerate laboratory investigation to confirm diagnosis.

Q.4. How you manage this patient? What can be the complications of galactosemia?

ANSWERS

A.1. This child most probably suffering from galactosemia.

- It is a rare, hereditary disorder of carbohydrate metabolism, inherited as an autosomal recessive genetic condition that affects the body's ability to convert galactose to glucose. This condition results due to deficiency of galactose-1-phosphate uridylyltransferase (GALT).
- **Figure 1.4.2** depicts the galactose metabolism.

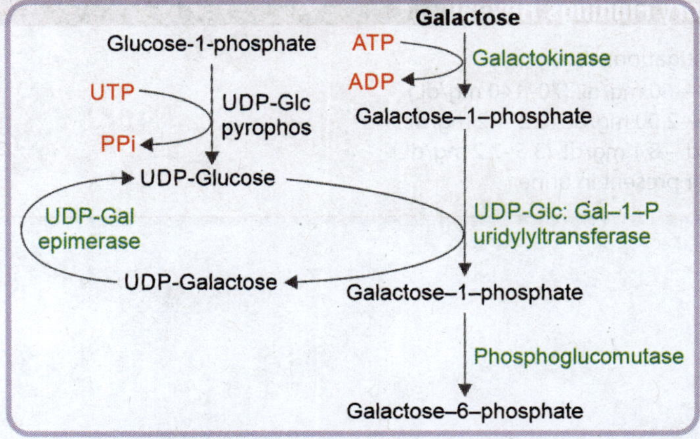

Fig. 1.4.2: Galactose metabolism.

A.2. Biochemical basis of clinical presentation of galactosemia are:

a. **Hypoglycemia:** Deficiency of key enzyme leads to accumulation of galactose-1-phosphate, this inhibits glycogen phosphorylase and prevents glycogenolysis, results in hypoglycemia.

b. **Hepatomegaly and jaundice:** Impaired galactose metabolism leads to accumulation of galactose in liver results in hepatomegaly, which further reduces bilirubin uptake and bilirubin conjugation.

c. **Kidney damage and aminoaciduria:** Galactose-1-phosphate may get deposited in renal tubules, producing tubular damage leading to generalized aminoaciduria.

d. **Cataract:** Enzyme deficiency leads to accumulation of galactose, it is reduced to galactitol (via polyol pathway). The accumulation of galactitol in the lens, because of osmotic effect absorbs water and result in cataract. Most of the cases are mild and transient, cataract changes are reversible only if galactose is withdrawn from food before the rupture of the cell membrane.

e. **Mental retardation:** The molecular and biochemical basis of mental retardation does not have a satisfactory explanation so far. Accumulation of galactitol with other toxic analytes could be a neurotoxin. Galactitol reduces the glutathione redox potential and causes cytotoxic effects.

A.3. Galactosemia classified in three forms (based on deficiency of enzyme):

Type 1: Classic galactosemia—galactose-1 phosphate uridylyltransferase (GALT) deficiency:, the most common and most severe form.

Type 2: Deficiency of galactose kinase (GALK).

Type 3: Deficiency of galactose-6-phosphate epimerase (GALE).

Laboratory investigation helpful in diagnosis of galactosemia.

A blood test will detect the reduced activity of associated enzymes and high levels of galactose (GALK deficiency) or high levels of galactose-1 phosphate (GALT deficiency)

Molecular genetic testing is also available to identify mutations in the *GALT* gene.

A.4. Management of galactosemia is based on early restriction of dietary galactose with calcium supplements is essential. This should be started within two to three weeks of age because any delay results in irreversible damage to tissues. Food restrictions—breast milk, cow's milk, casein should be restricted promptly. Child should switched to soy-based formula.

If child comes with mature cataract which is too dense or mature, it requires surgical removal.

Development delay like apraxia (inability to perform task), dysarthria (difficulty in speech articulation) require specialized training like speech therapy.

Galactosemia patients face wide variety of complications as depicted in **Figure 1.4.3**.

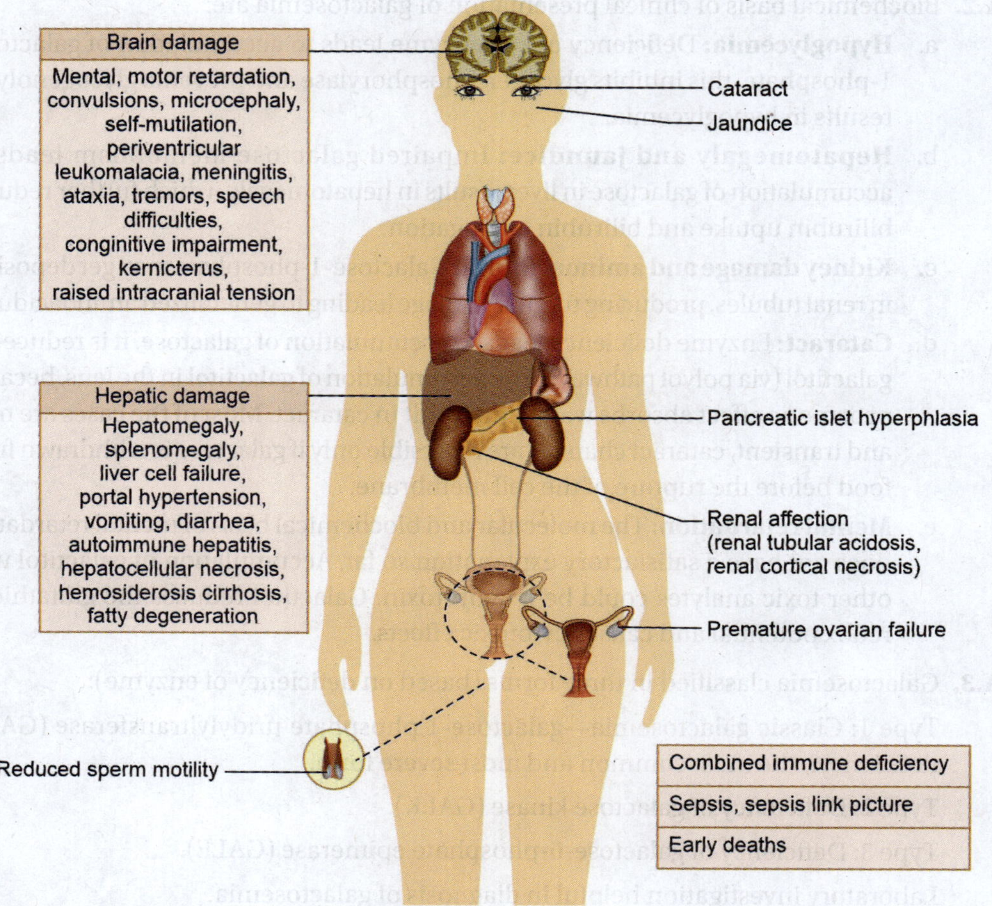

Fig. 1.4.3: Complications of galactosemia.

BIBLIOGRAPHY

1. Berry GT. Classic Galactosemia and Clinical Variant Galactosemia. 2000 Feb 4 [Updated 2021 Mar 11]. In: Adam MP, Everman DB, Mirzaa GM, et al., (Eds). Gene Reviews® [Internet]. Seattle (WA): University of Washington, Seattle; 1993-2022. Available from: https://www.ncbi.nlm.nih.gov/books/NBK1518/
2. Pasquali M, Yu C, Coffee B. Laboratory diagnosis of galactosemia: a technical standard and guideline of the American College of Medical Genetics and Genomics (ACMG). Genet Med. 2018;20(1):3-11.

Case 1.5

Glycogen Storage Disease

COMPETENCY

❖ **BC3.5:** Discuss the mechanism and significance of blood glucose regulation (glucose homeostasis) in health and disease. Describe the types, biochemical changes, complications and laboratory investigations related to diabetes and other carbohydrate metal disorders

Case Scenario

A 3-month-old infant presented to the emergency with seizure. She has doll like face, chubby cheeks and thin limbs. Predominant hepatomegaly with mild splenomegaly. Liver transaminases are normal despite of hepatomegaly. Hypoglycemia, hyperuricemia with lactic acidosis is present. The infant was previously prescribed with frequent meals.

QUESTIONS

Q.1. What would be the probable diagnosis? Describe the biochemical basis of this condition.

Q.2. Explain biochemical basis of sign and symptoms of this condition.

Q.3. Enumerate laboratory investigation to confirm diagnosis.

Q.4. How you manage this patient? Enlist the other possible differential diagnosis of the patients with similar clinical findings.

ANSWERS

A.1. Child most probably suffering from Von Gierke disease also known as glycogen storage disease (GSD) type 1, is an autosomal recessive disease in which there is an inability to cleave glycogen to glucose because of a glucose-6-phosphatase deficiency.

A.2. Biochemical basis of sign and symptom (**Fig. 1.5.1**).

Hypoglycemia

Deficiency of enzyme glucose-6-phosphatase causes accumulation of glucose-6-phosphate, resulting in profound hypoglycemia, which may result as repeated loss of consciousness, tremors and seizures. Long-term low blood sugar can lead to delayed growth and development and muscle weakness.

- Hypoglycemia leads to seizure, coma, intellectual disability, cognitive impairement, delayed growth and development
- Liver and kidney enlargement: Due to accumulation of glycogen
- Hyperuricemia
- Hyperlipidemia (leads to xanthoma)
- Typically doll-like faces with fat cheeks and relatively thin extremities
- Short stature, hypotonia
- Recurrent infections
- Epistaxis infections
- Epistaxis (impaired platelet function)

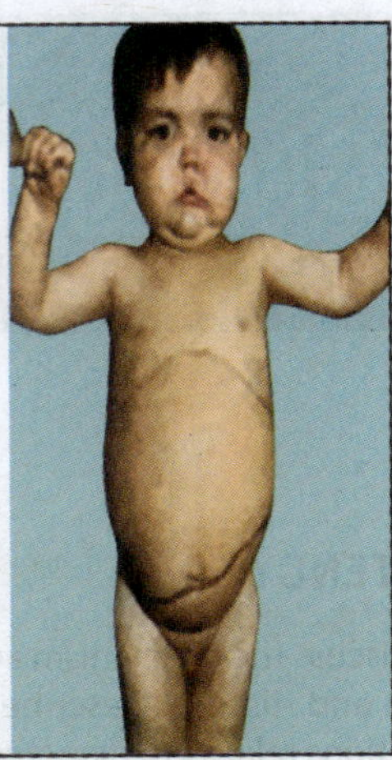

Fig. 1.5.1: Clinical presentation of glycogen storage disorder type 1.

Lactic Acidosis

Accumulation of glucose-6-phosphate, that may enter in glycolysis leads to formation of excessive pyruvate and its reduction to lactic acid.

Hyperuricemia

Glucose-6-phosphate also enters in HMP shunt pathway and causes excess formation of ribose sugar, that is used in nucleic acid formation. Breakdown of nucleic acid causes increase production of uric acid resulting in hyperuricemia.

A.3. GSD type I is diagnosed by laboratory tests that indicate abnormal levels of glucose, lactate, uric acid, triglycerides, and cholesterol.

Liver biopsy can also be used to prove specific enzyme deficiency for GSD Ia.

Molecular genetic testing for mutation analysis and specific genes detection to confirm a diagnosis.

A.4. GSD type I is treated with a special diet in order to maintain normal glucose levels, prevent hypoglycemia and maximize growth and development. Frequent small servings of carbohydrates must be maintained during the day and night throughout the life.

Other glycogen storage disorders given in **Table 1.5.1**, which can be a choice in differential diagnosis of above clinical presentation.

Table 1.5.1: Glycogen storage disorders.

Type	*Defective enzyme*	*Organ affected*	*Glycogen in the affected organ*	*Clinical features*
I. Von Gierke	Glucose-6-phosphatase or transport system	Liver and kidney	Increased amount; normal structure	Massive enlargement of the liver. Failure to thrive. Severe hypoglycemia, ketosis, hyperuricemia, hyperlipemia

Contd...

Contd...

Type	*Defective enzyme*	*Organ affected*	*Glycogen in the affected organ*	*Clinical features*
II. Pompe	α -l,4-Glucosidase (lysosomal)	All organs	Massive increase in amount; normal structure	Cardiorespiratory failure causes death, usually before age 2.
III. Cori	Amylo-1,6-glucosidase (debranching enzyme)	Muscle and liver	Increased amount; short outer branches	Like type I, but milder course.
IV. Andersen	Branching enzyme (α-l,4 → α-l,6)	Liver and spleen	Normal amount; very long outer branches	Progressive cirrhosis of the liver. Liver failure causes death, usually before age 2
V. McArdle	Phosphorylase	Muscle	Moderately increased amount; normal structure	Limited ability to perform strenuous exercise because of painful muscle cramps. Otherwise patient is normal and well developed
IV. Hers	Phosphorylase	Liver	Increased amount	Like type I, but milder course
VII.	Phosphofructokinase	Muscle	Increased amount; normal structure	Like type V
VIII.	Phosphorylase kinase	Liver	Increased amount; normal structure	Mild liver enlargement. Mild hypoglycemia

BIBLIOGRAPHY

1. Avalos S, Mejia RE, Banegas E, Salinas C, Gutierrez L, Fajardo M, Galo S, Pinto A, Mejia A, Fontecha G. G6PD deficiency, primaquine treatment, and risk of haemolysis in malaria-infected patients. Malar J. 2018;17(1):415.
2. Richardson SR, O'Malley GF. Glucose-6-Phosphate Dehydrogenase Deficiency. [Updated 2022 Sep 26]. In: StatPearls [Internet]. Treasure Island (FL): StatPearls Publishing; 2022 Jan. Available from: https://www.ncbi.nlm.nih.gov/books/NBK470315/

Case 1.6

Lactose intolerance

COMPETENCY

- **BC3.2:** Describe the digestion, absorption and transport of carbohydrates from food along with its disorders

Integration with Pediatrics

- **PE23.4:** Define diarrhea (acute diarrhea, chronic diarrhea, persistent diarrhea). Discuss etiology, risk factors, clinical features, complications, investigations and treatment (according to WHO guidelines) of acute gastroenteritis

Case Scenario

A 20-year-old man presents at the medical OPD with complains of abdominal pain, diarrhea and muscle cramps **(Fig. 1.6.1)**. From the case history, it appears that he had consumed a large quantity of milk and other dairy product for three days on a festive occasion. The house surgeon, who examined him (after ruling out other causes of acute abdomen), advised him to avoid milk, however advice to take curd. The patient followed this advice and became normal in 2 days.

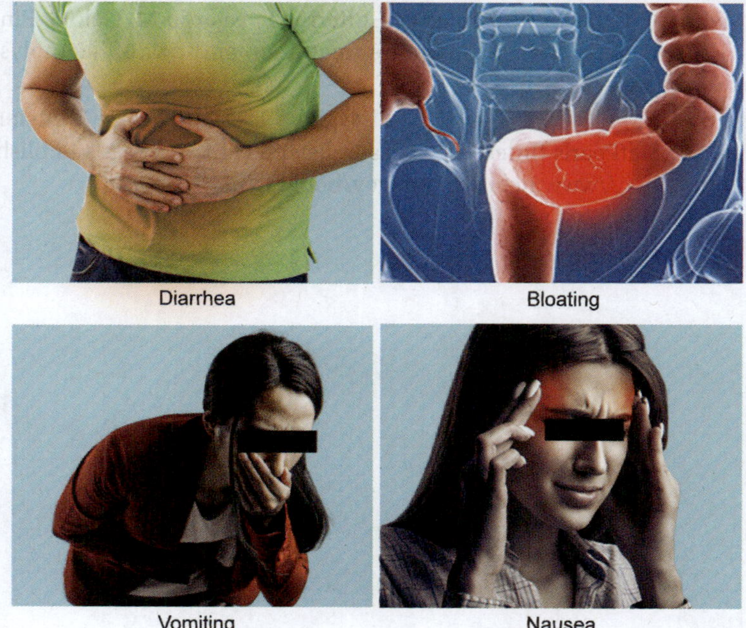

Fig. 1.6.1: Clinical presentation of lactose intolerance.

QUESTIONS

Q.1. What is the probable diagnosis? What are the causes for the above condition?

Q.2. Explain the biochemical basis of the sign and symptoms of this disorder.

Q.3. How will you diagnose this case?

Q.4. What treatments will you advice to the patient? Explain the rationale behind the treatment.

ANSWERS

A.1. Patient is suffering from lactose intolerance.

This is due to deficiency of lactase enzyme (digestive disaccharidase/beta galactosidase). This clinical condition affects approximately 70% of world population.

There are three main types of lactose intolerance:

A. Primary lactose intolerance (normal result of aging): This is the most common type of lactose intolerance. Most people are born with enough lactase. The amount of lactase a person makes may decrease over time. This is because as people age, they eat a more diverse diet and rely less on milk. The decline in lactase is gradual. This type of lactose intolerance is more common in people with Asian, African, and Hispanic ancestry.

B. Secondary lactose intolerance (due to illness or injury): Intestinal diseases such as celiac disease rota virus infection and inflammatory bowel disease (IBD), a surgery, or an injury to your small intestine can also cause lactose intolerance. Lactase levels may be restored if the underlying disorder is treated.

C. Congenital or developmental lactose intolerance:

   i. In very rare cases, lactose intolerance is inherited. A defective gene can be transmitted from the parents to a child, resulting in the complete absence of lactase in the child. This is referred to as congenital lactose intolerance.

   ii. Occasionally, a type of lactose intolerance called developmental lactose intolerance occurs when a baby is born prematurely. This is because lactase production in the baby begins later in the pregnancy, after at least 34 weeks.

A.2. Biochemical basis of signs and symptoms:

Lactose sugar is not metabolized due to deficiency of lactase, results in accumulation of the lactose in the intestine, this undigested and unabsorbed lactose is osmotically active and draws fluid on intestinal lumen resulting in diarrhea, this lactose undergo bacterial degradation and produce hydrogen(H_2), carbon dioxide (CO_2) and methane (CH_4) which results in flatulence **(Fig. 1.6.2)**. Bloating and distension in the abdomen.

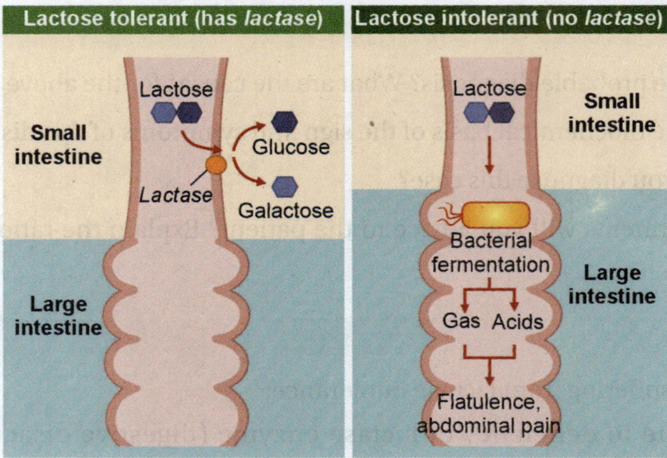

Fig. 1.6.2: Intestinal symptoms in lactose intolerance.

A.3. Diagnosis of lactose intolerance can be done by following test:

- **Hydrogen breath test:** After taking a liquid that contains high levels of lactose, amount of hydrogen in breath measured at regular intervals. Breathing out too much hydrogen indicates that patient isn't fully digesting and absorbing lactose.
- **Lactose tolerance test:** Two hours after drinking a liquid that contains high levels of lactose, patient undergo blood tests to measure the amount of glucose in bloodstream. If glucose level does not rise, it means body isn›t properly digesting and absorbing the lactose-filled drink.
- In infant stool pH (typically below 5.5 and presence of reducing sugar in stool) is indirect test for lactose intolerance.

A.4. Patient will be advised to withdraw the intake of milk temporarily and as lactase is an inducible enzyme, body will get time to synthesize the enzyme. Curd and Yoghurt are rich in bacteria that contain high levels of the lactase enzyme and this enzyme acts in the intestine to help digest the lactose **(Fig. 1.6.3)**.

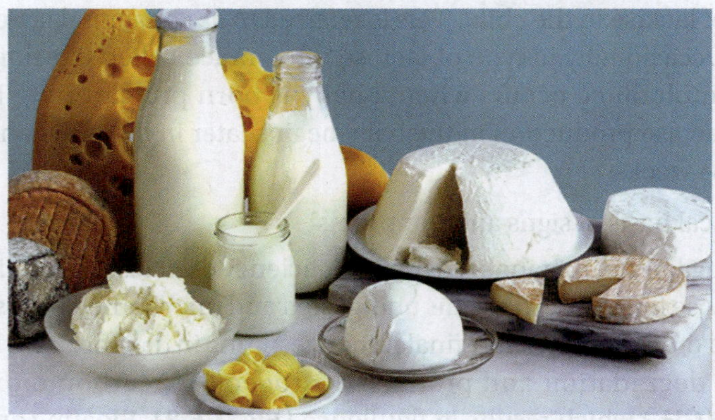

Fig. 1.6.3: Milk and milk products rich in lactose.

BIBLIOGRAPHY

1. Malik TF, Panuganti KK. Lactose Intolerance. [Updated 2022 May 16]. In: StatPearls [Internet]. Treasure Island (FL): StatPearls Publishing; 2022 Jan-. Available from: https://www.ncbi.nlm.nih.gov/books/NBK532285/
2. Szilagyi A, Ishayek N. Lactose Intolerance, Dairy Avoidance, and Treatment Options. Nutrients. 2018;10(12):1994.

Case 1.7

Mucopolysaccharidosis

COMPETENCY

- **BC6.1:** Enumerate the functions and components of the extracellular matrix (ECM)
- **BC6.2:** Discuss the involvement of ECM components in health and disease

Case Scenario

An 8-year-old female patient presents with complaints of respiratory distress, massive abdominal distension, and generalized body swelling. Her parents reveal developmental milestones slowed down, with gradual mental decline expressed in terms of lost physical skills. And multiple joint stiffness and that the patient was having difficulty in walking for last few years and was unable to walk in the last year of her life. In the past few years, the patient had multiple chest infections. Physical examination revealed coarse facial features, low set ears, depressed nasal bridge, rotated legs, short neck, distended abdomen, thick short claw-like hands, umbilical hernia, and kyphosis.

QUESTIONS

Q.1. What would be the probable diagnosis? Describe the biochemical basis of this condition.

Q.2. How you reach on confirm diagnosis?

Q.3. What is the management of this case?

ANSWERS

A.1. Patient most probably suffering from mucopolysaccharidosis.

Mucopolysaccharidosis (MPS) are a group of genetic metabolic disorders due to the absence or malfunctioning of specific enzymes required to process molecules called glycosaminoglycans. MPS is a part of the lysosomal storage disorders family. These disorders are caused by malfunctioning of lysosomes. Clinical pesentations of mucopolysaccharidosis is summarized in **Figure 1.7.1.**

Biochemical basis of disease

In MPS, there is deficiencies of enzymes needed to break down glycosaminoglycans. This leads to glycosaminoglycan build up in the cells **(Table 1.7.1)**, blood and

- **CNS:** Congitive impairment, behavioral problems, developmental delay and mental retardation
- **Skeletal:** Dysplasia and abnormal bone size, facial feature like flat nasal bridge and thick lips, short torso
- **Eyes:** Corneal opacities, retinopathies, glaucoma
- **Ears:** Recurrent cold, otitis, hearing loss
- **Others:** Enlarged organs like heart, liver and spleen, heart and respiratory disease

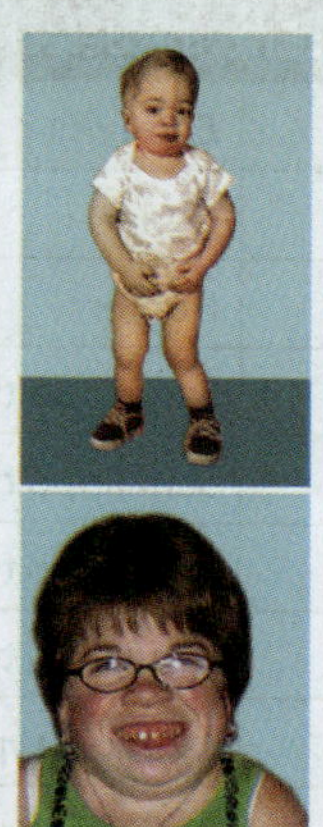

Fig. 1.7.1: Clinical presentation of mucopolysaccharidosis.

Table 1.7.1: Accumulation of GAG in different mucopolysaccharidosis.

Type	*Name of the syndrome*	*GAG accumulated*
MPS Type I	Hurler's syndrome/Scheie syndrome	Dermatan, heparan sulfate
MPS Type II	Hunter's syndrome	Dermatan, heparan sulfate
MPS Type III	Sanfilippo syndrome	Heparan sulfate
MPS Type IV	Morquio syndrome	Keratan sulfate, chondroitin sulfate
MPS Type VI	Maroteaux-Lamy syndrome	Dermatan, chondroitin sulfate
MPS Type VII	Sly syndrome	Dermatan/heparan chondroitin sulfate
MPS Type IX	Natowicz syndrome	Hyaluronan

Source: National Organization for Rare Disorders (NORD).
(MPS: mucopolysaccharidosis; GAG: glycosaminoglycan)

connective tissue and consequent cellular damage. The cellular damage manifests as symptoms like abnormal facial features and appearance, impaired physical ability, organ malfunctioning and in some cases, cognitive impairments and developmental delay.

A.2. Diagnosis of MPS can be done on the basis of:

a. Urine tests indicate the presence of excess mucopolysaccharides.
b. Enzyme assays where cultured cells or blood is tested for enzyme deficiencies is also diagnostic of the specific type of mucopolysaccharidoses (**Table 1.7.2**).
c. Genetic testing is available to detect carriers of the gene. Prenatal diagnosis is also available to detect the presence of MPS in the fetus.

Table 1.7.2: Enzyme defect in different mucopolysaccharidosis.

MPS type	*Eponym*	*Enzyme defect*
I	Hurler	α-L-iduronidase
II	Hunter	Iduronate 2-sulfatase
III-A	Sanfilippo type A	Heparan N-sulfatase
III-B	Sanfilippo type B	α-N-acetylglucosaminidase
III-C	Sanfilippo type C	Acetyl-CoA: α-glucosaminide N-acetyltransferase
III-D	Sanfilippo type C	N-acetylglucosamine-6-sulfatase
III-A	Morquio type A	Galactose 6-sulfatase
IV-B	Morquio type B	β-galactosidase
VI	Maroteaux-Lamy	N-acetylgalactosamine 4-sulfatase
VII	Sly	β-glucuronidase

A.3. There is no permanent cure for MPS and treatment is symptomatic.

MPS is treated on a case-to-case basis in providing support for patients. Nutritional supplements may be given to maintain strength.

Enzyme replacement therapy (ERT) is being used for MPS I, MPS II and MPS VI. This is helpful in reducing pain and neurological symptoms.

Bone marrow transplant (BMT) and umbilical cord blood transplant (UCBT) have not been very successful treating MPS.

BIBLIOGRAPHY

1. https://rarediseases.org/rare-diseases/mucopolysaccharidoses/
2. https://www.mpsreference.com.au/management-and-treatment-of-mps/mps-vi-maroteaux-lamy-syndrome/
3. Muenzer J. Overview of the mucopolysaccharidoses. Rheumatology. 2011;50(Suppl 5): v4–v12.

GIVE REASONS WHY

Q.1. Deficiency of G6PD in red blood cells may lead to hemolysis.

Ans. G6PD activity keeps the oxidative stress of RBC reduced. It is the key regulating enzyme of HMP shunt pathway which is a minor metabolic pathway of glucose metabolism, where pentose and NADPH is produced from glucose. NADPH is a major reducing agent in RBCs that generates reduced glutathione, essential for prevention of hemolysis due to free radical attack.

Q.2. Insulin therapy in diabetic ketoacidosis leads to hypokalemia.

Ans. In patients of DKA, deficiency of potassium is expected due to osmotic diuresis, emesis, and secondary hyperaldosteronism, though pretreatment serum potassium levels are usually not low due to the extracellular shift of potassium that occurs with acidosis and insulin deficiency. As soon as insulin treatment is initiated, potassium shifts intracellularly and serum levels decline. Intravenous potassium replacement is the standard of care in treatment of DKA to prevent the potential consequences of hypokalemia including cardiac arrhythmias and respiratory failure.

Q.3. Uronic acid pathway play important role in metabolism of Xenobiotics.

Ans. Xenobiotic is a term used to describe chemical substances that not naturally produced / foreign to humans. Metabolic pathways involve in removal of such xenobiotic substance are collectively known as Xenobiotics. Uronic acid pathway results in formation of UDP glucuronic acid, which is an active form of glucuronic acid. UPP glucuronic acid is used for conjugation of various drugs and makes them water soluble and easily excretable.

Q.4. Patients with diabetic ketoacidosis have Kussmaul breathing.

Ans. Kussmaul breathing (rapid breathing) is a type of respiratory compensatory mechanism by which metabolic acidosis is compensated by releasing CO_2 (acidic in nature) through hyperventilation and maintains the blood pH around normal (7.4).

Q.5. Intake of dietary fibers in diets leads to decrease serum cholesterol.

Ans. High dietary fiber content increases the motility of bowels and reduces the reabsorption of bile salts, that is how indirectly reduce absorption of the cholesterol.

Q.6. Increase activity of Rapoport-Luebering shunt in high altitude.

Ans. Rapoport-Luebering shunt also known as bisphosphoglycerate shunt, through which enzyme mutase convert 1,3 bisphosphoglycerate to 2,3 bisphosphoglycerate. It takes place in RBC 2,3 BPG combines with hemoglobin and reduces its affinity towards oxygen. So in hypoxic conditions like in high altitude the formation of 2,3 BPG increase through above shunt and causes increase release of oxygen from hemoglobin.

Q.7. Deficiency of thiamine leads to decrease activity of PDH (pyruvate dehydrogenase complex).

Ans. PDH is a complex enzyme system, which requires water soluble vitamins for its functioning. One of them is thiamine, so not only deficiency of thiamine but deficiency of lipoic acid , CoA (pantothenic acid) , FAD (riboflavin) and (niacin) NAD^+ can cause decrease activity of PDH complex.

Q.8. Cataract formation is in uncontrolled diabetes.

Ans. High level of glucose enhances glucose concentration in lens also, where it is reduced to sorbitol. Once sorbitol is synthesized it cannot come out from the cells of lens. Sorbitol is osmotically active. Its accumulation in lens leads to increase absorption of water in the cells of lens causes opacity.

Q.9. Women with gestational diabetes mellitus (GDM) is associated with increased weight of child.

Ans. In GDM, hyperglycemia of maternal blood stimulates secretion of excess insulin in fetus causing excessive fetal growth and birth weight child.

Q.10. Alimentary glycosuria occurs in hyperthyroidism.

Ans. Hyperthyroidism promotes rapid absorption of glucose from intestine. This will result in abrupt rise in glucose after food intake, however of fasting and postprandial glucose levels remain within normal range. This is known as alimentary glycosuria. This is also seen in gastrectomy.

Q.11. Impaired incretin system is associated with diabetes mellitus.

Ans. Incretins are a kind of protein hormones whose functions include the modulation of glucose metabolism by stimulating the release of insulin by the β cells and, at the same time, inhibiting the release of glucagon by pancreatic α cells. The incretin effect is defined as the increased stimulation of insulin secretion elicited by oral as compared with intravenous administration of glucose. There are 2 types of incretin hormones which have been identified, i.e., glucose dependent insulinotropic polypeptide (GIP) and glucagon-like peptide-1 (GLP-1). Defect in synthesis and release of these hormones cause deficiency of insulin, which results in diabetes mellitus.

Q.12. Thiamine deficiency leads to decrease of HMP shunt pathway.

Ans. One of the enzyme (transketolase) of HMP shunt pathway is TPP (thiamine pyrophosphate) dependent, so thiamine deficiency leads to decrease activity of transketolase and further to HMP shunt.

Q.13. Insulin is also known as hormone of anabolism.

Ans. Insulin promotes glycogenesis, lipogenesis, protein synthesis and cell replication. So it is also known as hormone of anabolism.

Q.14. Glycogenolysis in muscle does not help in regulation of blood glucose.

Ans. As the end product of glycogenolysis is glucose-1-PO_4 which after isomerization forms glucose-6-PO_4. Muscle cell are deficient of glucose-6 phosphatase, which is required to release glucose in the blood from glucose-6-PO_4.

Q.15. In anaerobic condition end product of glycolysis is lactic acid.

Ans. In anaerobic condition, the further process of pyruvate is not done through TCA cycle. At the same time to make the glycolysis continue to get whatever ATPs are generated through anaerobic glycolysis, there is a need to regenerate NAD^+. That can be done if pyruvate reduces into lactic acid.

Q.16. Vitamin-C cannot be synthesized in human beings.

Ans. In glucuronic acid pathway one intermediate compound is synthesized that is known as L-gulonic acid, which further metabolized by two metabolic pathways. In first pathway it will finally converted into xylitol. In second pathway enzyme gulonolactone oxidase is needed to synthesize vitamin-C and this enzyme is absent in human being that's why vitamin-C cannot be synthesized.

Section 2

Protein Metabolism

- **Case 2.1:** Albinism
- **Case 2.2:** Alkaptonuria
- **Case 2.3:** Maple Syrup Urine Disease
- **Case 2.4:** Multiple Myeloma
- **Case 2.5:** Phenylketonuria
- **Case 2.6:** Protein-Energy Malnutrition
- **Case 2.7:** Urea Cycle Disorders

Give Reasons Why

Case 2.1

Albinism

COMPETENCY

❖ **BC5.7:** Describe the specialized products formed from the amino acids Glycine, Phenylalanine, Tyrosine, Tryptophan, and Methionine, branched chain amino acids and Arginine and the inborn errors associated with them. Discuss newborn screening

Case Scenario

A 13-year-old boy, with total depigmentation of the skin, hair, and iris visited eye hospital for reduced visual acuity. Ophthalmologic examination revealed characteristic iris depigmentation and translucency, retinal depigmentation, foveal hypoplasia, misrouting of the optic nerve fibers, prominent photophobia, and nystagmus. He had normal mental development. Through examination was done to exclude other congenital deformities.

QUESTIONS

Q.1. What is the most probable diagnosis of this patient? What is the other differential diagnosis of this patient?

Q.2. Explain biochemical basis to explain clinical presentation of this patients.

Q.3. What is the management of this patient?

ANSWERS

A.1. Patient is most probably suffering from albinism. Albinism, from the Latin *albus*, meaning "white," is a group of heritable conditions associated with decreased or absent melanin in ectoderm-derived tissues (most notably the skin, hair, and eyes) (**Fig. 2.1.1**). Patients with albinism are particularly susceptible to solar damage, and these patients must utilize lifelong sun protection precautions. In albinism exact number of melanocytes in the skin are preserved. Other clinical condition like piebaldism and vitiligo, where melanocytes are absent also present in similar pattern.

A.2. Melanocytes which are ectodermal in origin migrate into the skin, eyes, hair, and inner ear during embryonic development. Melanosomes which is present in melanocytes responsible for production of melanin. The two most common forms of melanin are eumelanin and pheomelanin. Eumelanin fills skin with black or brown coloration and plays a role in protecting the skin against ultraviolet radiation B (UVB) damage

- White hair and very light-colored skin
- Extreme nearsightedness or farsightedness
- Sensitivity to light (photophobia)
- Abnormal curvature of the front surface of the eye or the lens inside the eye (astigmatism), which causes blurred vision
- Abnormal development of the retina, resulting in reduced vision
- Nystagmus (rapid, involuntary back-and-forth movement of the eyes)
- Strabismus (inability of both eyes to stay directed at the same point)

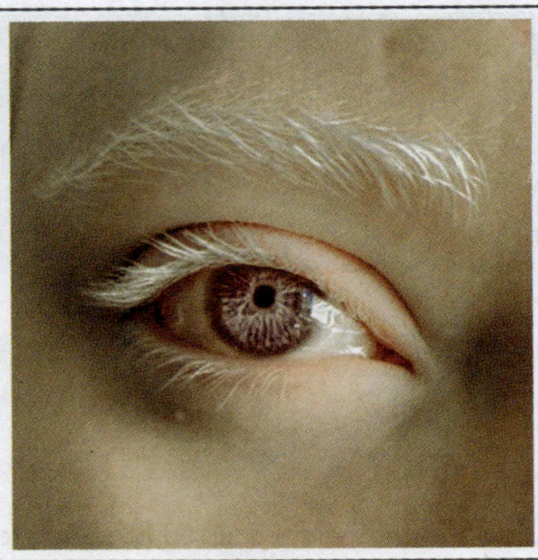

Fig. 2.1.1: Clinical presentation of albinism.

by absorbing and dissipating the rays and their carcinogenic DNA cross-linking effects. Pheomelanin is not UV protective and responsible for red or blond hair and light-colored, ruddy skin.

Enzyme tyrosinase is responsible in formation of eumelanin synthesis from DOPA. Mutations in the tyrosinase gene, leads to complete loss of the ability to produce eumelanin (**Fig. 2.1.2**).

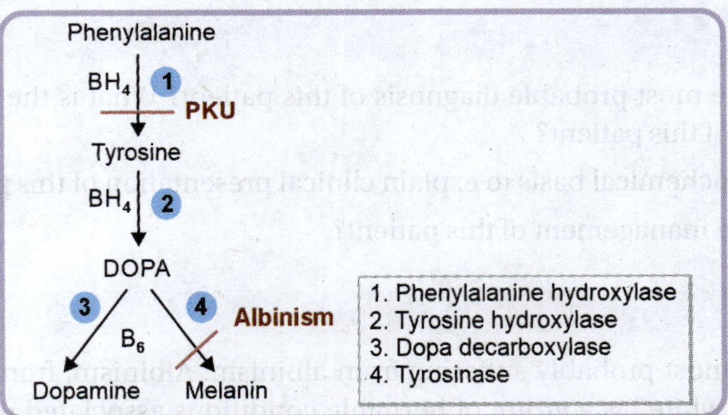

Fig. 2.1.2: Metabolic enzymes in phenylalanine metabolism.

The two significant results of hypomelanosis can be divided into dermatological and ophthalmologic consequences:

1. **Dermatological**: Increased risk of sun-damage (solar lentigines, actinic keratoses, solar erythema) and UV-associated malignancies (especially squamous cell carcinomas).
2. **Ophthalmological:** Melanin acts as an inducer and organizer of formation of the fovea, optic nerves, optic tracts, and visual cortex, in utero. Complete absence or even partial melanin deficiency leads to ocular structure deformity and optic

tract malformation which results in irreversible intraocular (refractive) and extraocular (oculomotor or nonrefractive) problems.

A.3. Management of patients can only be done by symptomatic treatment. Lifelong sun protection, avoidance of prolonged UV light exposure (sun, tanning beds) and avoidance of medications that increase photosensitivity.

Photophobia can be managed with dark lensed glasses.

Additional protection can be enlisted with the use of protective clothing and eyewear, hats, UPF-labelled clothing, long-sleeves, long pants, collared shirts, socks.

Management of eye abnormalities including correction of refractive errors, eye muscle surgery can improve ocular alignment.

Genetics consultation before childbearing years is beneficial to parents of albino children considering future offspring, the patient with albinism and their siblings.

BIBLIOGRAPHY

1. Federico JR, Krishnamurthy K. Albinism. [Updated 2022 Aug 22]. In: StatPearls [Internet]. Treasure Island (FL): StatPearls Publishing; 2022. Available from: https://www.ncbi.nlm.nih.gov/books/NBK519018/
2. King RA, Summers CG. Albinism. Dermatol Clin. 1988;6(2):217-28.
3. Oetting WS, King RA. Molecular basis of albinism: mutations and polymorphisms of pigmentation genes associated with albinism. Hum Mutat. 1999;13(2):99-115.

Case 2.2

Alkaptonuria

COMPETENCY

❖ **BC5.7:** Describe the specialized products formed from the amino acids Glycine, Phenylalanine, Tyrosine, Tryptophan, and Methionine, branched chain amino acids and Arginine and the inborn errors associated with them. Discuss newborn screening

Case Scenario

A 44-year-old woman came to the dermatology clinic with the complain of development of grey pigmentation of the external ear since last month. Also she had a rounded papule on the right cheek with dotted black pigmentation which was sent for histopathological examination. It showed yellow-brown and irregular-shaped fibers. Her history reveals darkening of urine on standing and narrowing and calcification of intervertebral spaces. Right-sided Achilles tendon rupture, and joint pain and stiffness for many years.

QUESTIONS

Q.1. What is the most probable diagnosis? Add a note on different clinical signs and symptoms of this disorder.

Q.2. Explain the biochemical basis for this clinical condition.

Q.3. How you can confirm your diagnosis?

Q.4. What is the management for this disorder?

ANSWERS

A.1. Lady is most probably suffering from alkaptonuria. It is an autosomal recessive metabolic disorder of amino acid metabolism phenylalanine and tyrosine.

Alkaptonuria: Clinical Signs and Symptoms (Fig. 2.2.1)

Outer ear: Bluish coloration of outer ear cartilage, more common after age 30, which may be accompanied by blackened coloration of earwax.

Ocular: Pigmentation of sclera, cornea, conjunctiva, eyelids, brownish coloration is common in the temporal and nasal corner of the sclera after age 40.

Skin: Brownish coloration in the malar and axillary regions, where there is a great number of sweat glands. There may be also papules and blackened blue vesicles in the palmar and plantar regions, due to friction of movements.

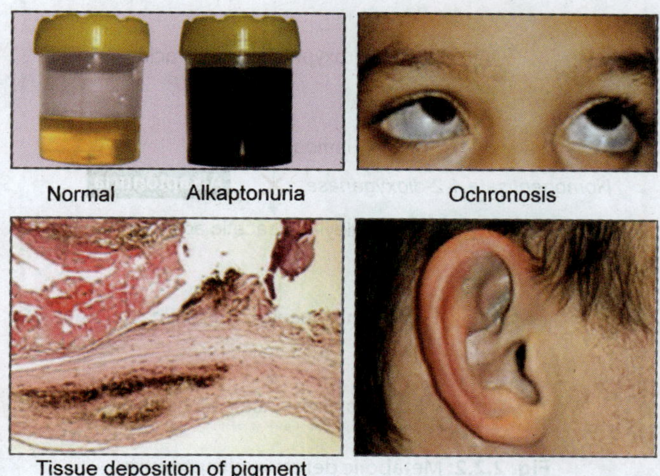

Fig. 2.2.1: Clinical presentation of alkaptonuria.

Genitourinary system: The initial symptom is the alteration of urine coloration, which is blackened in environmental air. It is predominant in males, and the prostate is frequently involved. Patients may have renal, prostatic lithiasis and other organs, such as gallbladder and salivary glands can also involed.

Cardiovascular system: Calcification of the aortic and mitral valve, besides deposition of pigment over valves, endocardium, aorta and coronary arteries. About 40% over 40–50 years of age will have some degree of cardiovascular involvement.

Skeletal system: Cases of arthropathy by ochronosis are common after 40 years of age, and sometimes surgeries for articulation substitution are needed. The large articulations, which receive a great load of stress are the most affected, such as—hip, knee, shoulders. In the lumbar column, there may be narrowing and calcification of intervertebral spaces. Rupture of ligaments and tendons.

A.2. Alkaptonuria is a rare inherited metabolic disorder characterized by blackening of urine on standing occurs due to deficiency of enzyme homogentisate oxidase in phenylalanine and tyrosine amino acid metabolism **(Fig. 2.2.2)**.

This lead to accumulation of homogentisic acid, which gets oxidized and produces blue black pigment (ochronotic pigment). Homogentisic acid in excess deposited mainly in cartilaginous tissue, mucous membranes, skin, bone surface and internal cardiac structures, as well as excreted in biological solutions (urine, sweat and semen). The main complications of alkaptonuria are valvular calcifications and osteoarthritis, mainly in the joints of the cervical spine, besides dark pigmentation of skin, cartilage, sclera and other connective tissues.

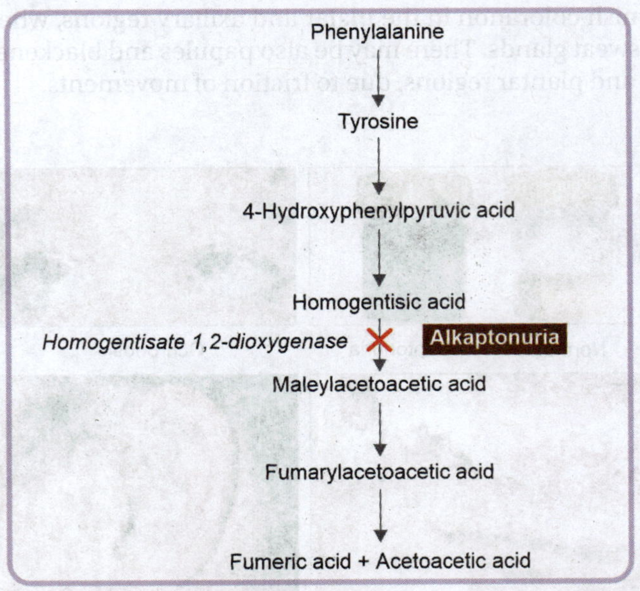

Fig. 2.2.2: Metabolic defect in alkaptonuria.

A.3. Diagnosis can be confirmed by:

Darkening of urine on standing due to elevated levels of homogentisic acid **(Fig. 2.2.3)** which can be detected by gas chromatography-mass spectrometry analysis. Supportive diagnosis can be made by histopathological examination of affected skin lesions.

Imaging techniques can be used to determine the presence and extent of joint and spinal disease or the involvement of the aortic or mitral valves. Computed tomography (CT) scan may be recommended to detect coronary artery calcification.

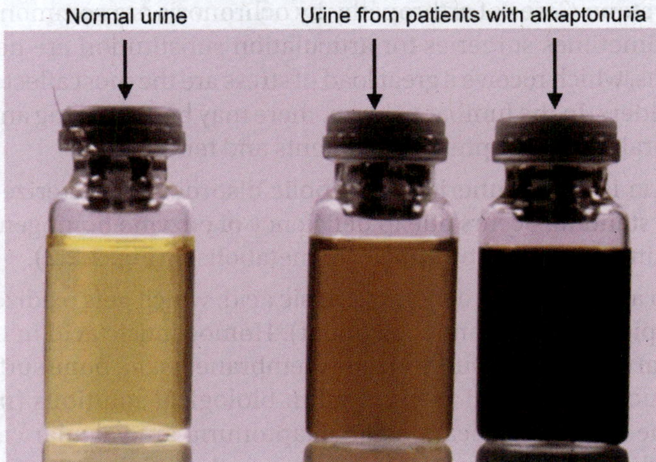

Fig. 2.2.3: Darkening of standing urine in patients of alkaptonuria.

A.4. Treatment of alkaptonuria is aimed at the specific symptoms that are present in each individual.

Anti-inflammatory medications (NSAIDs) for joint pain: Physical and occupational therapy, which can help maintain the strength and flexibility of muscles and joints.

Dietary restrictions have generally proven ineffective, though high-doses of vitamin C have also been used to treat alkaptonuria because it hinders the accumulation and deposition of homogentisic acid.

Activities that place significant physical stress to the spine and joints such as high impact sports or heavy manual labor should be avoided.

Investigational therapy: FDA approved **nitisinone** was shown to significantly reduce accumulations of homogentisic acid in individuals with alkaptonuria.

BIBLIOGRAPHY

1. Mistry JB, Bukhari M, Taylor AM. Alkaptonuria. Rare Dis. 2013;1:e27475.
2. Peker E, Yonden Z, Sogut S. From darkening urine to early diagnosis of alkaptonuria. Indian J Dermatol Venereol Leprol. 2008;74:700.

Case 2.3

Maple Syrup Urine Disease

COMPETENCY

❖ **BC5.7:** Describe the specialized products formed from the amino acids Glycine, Phenylalanine, Tyrosine, Tryptophan, and Methionine, branched chain amino acids and Arginine and the inborn errors associated with them. Discuss newborn screening

Case Scenario

A 1-week-old female infant presents with irritability, hypertonicity, high-pitched cry, and sleepiness. Baby was born at term after an uneventful normal vaginal delivery.

Laboratory investigations reveals metabolic acidosis, ketosis, and mild hyperammonemia. Baby's urine give a characteristic fruity/burnt sugar odor. Plasma and urine showed elevated levels of branched chain amino acids.

QUESTIONS

Q.1. What is the most probable diagnosis? What biochemical defect is present in this disorder?

Q.2. Explain the biochemical basis of these clinical signs and symptoms.

Q.3. Enumerate the laboratory tests to confirm the diagnosis.

Q.4. How will you manage the above condition?

ANSWERS

A.1. Biochemical basis of clinical presentation:

Deficiency of branched-chain alpha-keto acid dehydrogenase enzyme result in accumulation of all three BCAAs, along with a number of their toxic by-products, (specifically their respective organic acids).

Accumulation of leucine is predominantly responsible for neurological symptoms and peculiar maple syrup odor is due to elevated levels of isoleucine. Clinical signs and symptoms are summarized in **Figure 2.3.1**.

- Sweet smelling urine and sweat
- Poor feeding or loss of appetite
- Weight loss, lack of energy
- Vomiting, irritability
- Breathing difficulties
- Increasing hypertonia and spasticity progressing to seizures and coma
- Episodic metabolic crisis/sudden or gradual recurrent metabolic decompensation

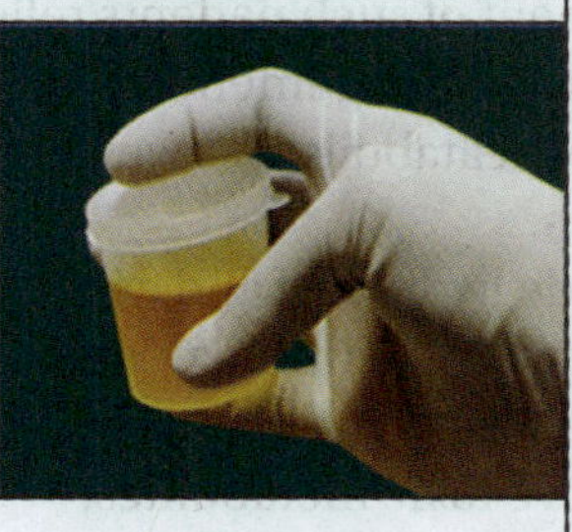

Fig. 2.3.1: Clinical presentation of maple syrup urine disease.

A.2. Most probable diagnosis is Maple Syrup Urine disease.

Maple syrup urine disease (MSUD) is a rare genetic disorder characterized by deficiency of an enzyme complex (branched-chain alpha-keto acid dehydrogenase) that is required to break down (metabolize) the three branched-chain amino acids (BCAAs) leucine, isoleucine and valine, in the body.

This enzyme complex helps in oxidative decarboxylation of branched chain amino acids (**Fig. 2.3.2**).

MSUD is classified in five clinical phenotype:

i. Classic
ii. Intermediate
iii. Intermittent
iv. Thiamine responsive
v. Dihydrolipoyl dehydrogenase deficient form

Classic type is most common and most severe type which presents with typical symptoms and neurological deterioration in first 3 to 4 days of birth.

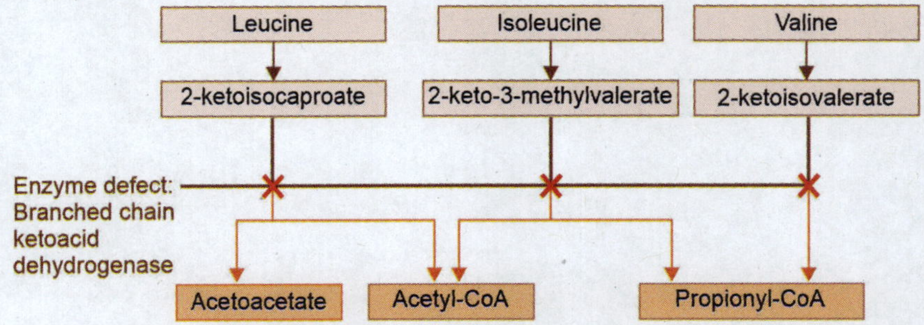

Fig. 2.3.2: Enzyme defect in maple syrup urine disease.

A.3. Laboratory tests to confirm the diagnosis:

a. Presence of branched chain amino acids in urine.
b. Rothera's test will be positive
c. Branched chain amino acids in blood >250 nmol/mL

A.4. Management of such patients relies on:

a. Dietary management by reducing BCAAs with adequate macronutrients to prevent catabolism as well to maintain plasma BCAAs within targeted treatment ranges.

b. Provide hydration and calorific support.

c. Correct and minimize any metabolic abnormalities and associated clinical sequelae.

d. Remove toxic metabolites.

BIBLIOGRAPHY

1. Blackburn PR, Gass JM, Vairo FPE, Farnham KM, Atwal HK, Macklin S et al. Maple syrup urine disease: mechanisms and management. Appl Clin Genet. 2017;10:57-66.
2. https://rarediseases.org/rare-diseases/maple-syrup-urine-disease/
3. Strauss KA, Puffenberger EG, Carson VJ. Maple Syrup Urine Disease. 2006 [Updated 2020]. In: Adam MP, Everman DB, Mirzaa GM, et al., editors. GeneReviews® [Internet]. Seattle (WA): University of Washington, Seattle; 1993-2022. Available from: https://www.ncbi.nlm.nih.gov/books/NBK1319/

Case 2.4

Multiple Myeloma

COMPETENCY

- **BC5.4:** Describe plasma proteins and their functions and brief overview of normal and abnormal electrophoretic pattern of serum proteins, acute phase protein
- **BC14.19:** Explain the basis and rationale of biochemical tests done and interpretation of laboratory results in the following conditions: Renal failure, Nephrotic syndrome

Integration with Medicine

- **GM13.1:** Describe the clinical epidemiology and inherited and modifiable risk factors for common malignancies in India

Case Scenario

A 55-year-old woman had a fall at home, multiple fractures were found on X-ray. She had 5-month history of fatigue and hip pain however she did not have other comorbidities.

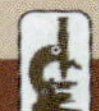

Laboratory Findings Reveal

- Hemoglobin: 10 g/dL
- Serum calcium: 11.5 (9–11 mg/dL)
- Serum total protein: 9 (6–8 g/dL)
- Serum albumin: 3 (3.5–5 g/dL)
- Serum globulin: 6 (2.5–3.5 g/dL)
- Serum protein electrophoresis reveals elevated gamma band

QUESTIONS

Q.1. What could be the probable diagnosis?

Q.2. Explain the biochemical basis for the symptoms of this clinical condition.

Q.3. How you confirm your diagnosis? Explain briefly electrophoretic pattern on above stated condition.

Q.4. What will be the management for the patient?

ANSWERS

A.1. Patient is most probably suffering from multiple myeloma. Multiple myeloma is a cancer of plasma cells. When B lymphocyte cells respond to an infection, they mature and change into plasma cells, which are found in the bone marrow and are an important part of the immune system. Plasma cells make the antibodies (also called immunoglobulins).

A.2. In multiple myeloma healthy plasma cells turn into abnormal cancerous cells that multiply and produce abnormal antibodies called M proteins, which is also known as Bence-Jones proteins, also referred to, myelomas proteins, paraproteins, and free immunoglobulin light chains.

This abnormal replication of B lymphocyte and accumulation of paraproteins responsible for clinical presentation of myeloma patients. Clinical signs and symptoms are summarized in **Figure 2.4.1**.

- Low blood counts (anemia, thrombocytopenia, leukopenia)
- Elevated blood calcium
- Blood hyperviscosity
- Renal failure
- Infection
- Bone pain, osteoporosis, fractures
- Spinal cord compression (back pain, numbness, muscle weakness, peripheral neuropathy)

Bone pain, especially in your spine
Loss of appetite
Fatigue
Weight loss
Frequent infections

Fig. 2.4.1: Clinical presentation of multiple myeloma.

A.3. Following tests may be used to diagnose multiple myeloma:

Blood and Urine Tests

1. **M protein:** Myeloma cells often secrete the antibody monoclonal immunoglobulin, known as M protein. M protein levels in a patient's blood and urine are used to determine the extent of the disease.
2. **Immunoglobulin:** Immunoglobulin levels in blood are measured to help check the amount of antibody levels in the blood. when the cancer protein level is up, the normal antibody levels are down.
3. **Light chains:** Light chain is found in the urine, it is called the Bence-Jones protein. These proteins are light chains of immunoglobulins. This protein has characteristic property to precipitate between 40 to 60 degrees centigrade, and dissolve when heated on high temperature and reprecipitate on 40 to 60 degree centigrade.
4. Serum albumin and serum beta-2 microglobulin (β2-M).
5. In gel electrophoresis, normal serum is separated into 5 bands. Gamma globulin has minimum mobility and remain at the site of origin. These globulins contain

immunoglobulins. Multiple myeloma results in formation of monoclonal origin of immunoglobulins, they appear as a sharp spike or M-band in electrophoresis **(Fig. 2.4.2)**.

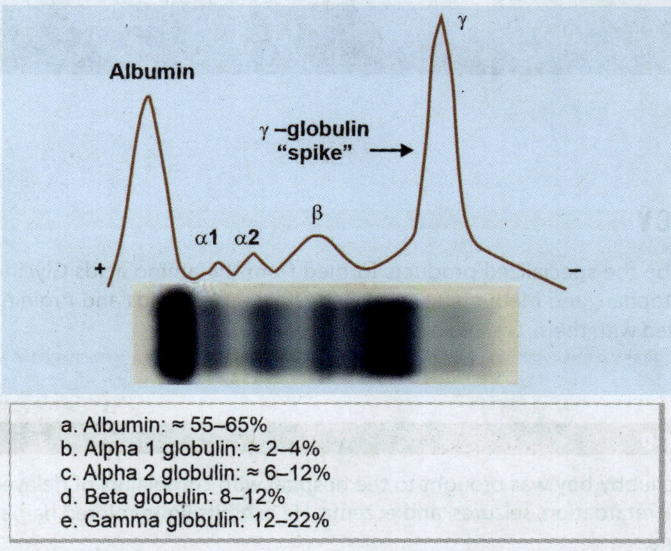

Fig. 2.4.2: Electrophoretic pattern of plasma proteins in multiple myeloma.

Imaging techniques

- X-ray, MRI, CT-scan, positron emission tomography (PET) or PET-CT scan.
- Bone marrow aspiration and biopsy
- Cytogenetics and fluorescence in situ hybridization (FISH)

A.4. Management

Treatment may be of two types:

a. Nonintensive—older/less fit patient
b. Intensive—younger patients

For both types patient need combination of anti-myeloma drugs like chemotherapy, steroids, thalidomide or bortezomib.

Stem cell transplant can be given in intensive treatment.

BIBLIOGRAPHY

1. https://rarediseases.org/rare-diseases/multiple-myeloma/
2. Rajkumar SV, Kumar S. Multiple Myeloma: Diagnosis and Treatment. Mayo Clin Proc. 2016; 91(1):101-19.

Case 2.5

Phenylketonuria

COMPETENCY

❖ **BC5.7:** Describe the specialized products formed from the amino acids Glycine, Phenylalanine, Tyrosine, Tryptophan, and Methionine, branched chain amino acids and Arginine and the inborn errors associated with them. Discuss newborn screening

Case Scenario

A 5-year old, fair, chubby boy was brought to the hospital with complaints of delayed developmental milestones, mental retardation, seizures, and eczema. He exhibits light-colored hair, skin and eyes and mousy odor in urine.

QUESTIONS

Q.1. **What is the most probable diagnosis? What biochemical defect is present in this disorder?**

Q.2. **Explain the biochemical basis of this clinical signs and symptoms.**

Q.3. **Enumerate the laboratory tests to confirm the diagnosis.**

Q.4. **How will you manage the above condition?**

ANSWERS

A.1. **Biochemical basis of clinical signs and symptoms are summarized in Figure 2.5.1.**

- Intellectual disability, psychiatric disorders
- Behavioral or social problems
- Seizures, shaking, or jerking movements in the arms and legs
- Delayed development, stunted or slow growth
- Skin rashes like eczema
- Small head size called microcephaly
- A musty odor in urine, breath, or skin
- Fair skin and blue eyes

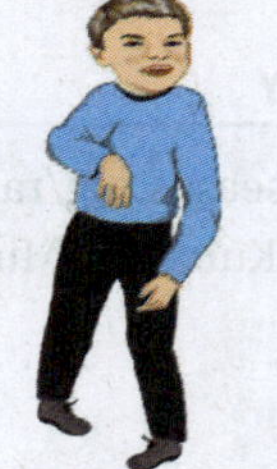

Fig. 2.5.1: Clinical presentation of phenylketonuria.

Mental retardation, hyperactivity and stunted growth, neurological manifestation

- Interference in synthesis of neurotransmitters (dopa, dopamine, catecholamines)
- Interference in synthesis of thyroxine.

Light color of the skin and blue color of eyes

- Interference in synthesis of melanin from tyrosine.

Mousy odor in breath and urine

- Abnormally elevated levels of phenyl ketones and phenyl acetate in blood and urine

A.2. Child most probably suffering from phenylketonuria. This is autosomal recessive disorder with the prevalence of 1:10,000. There is a defect in metabolic pathway of phenylalanine due to deficiency of phenylalanine hydroxylase (classical-type 1), niacin and tetrahydrobiopterin (**Fig. 2.5.2**).

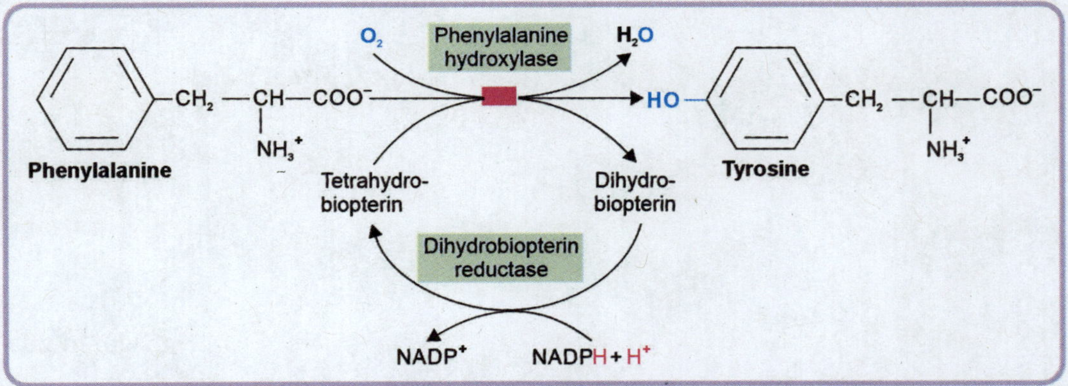

Fig. 2.5.2: Enzyme defects in phenylketonuria.

As phenylalanine cannot be metabolized to tyrosine, it enters into alternate pathways to form other metabolites like phenylpyruvate, phenyllactate, phenyl acetate and phenylacetylglutamine. The term **phenylketonuria** is derived because of excretion of these metabolites in urine and **mousy odor** is due to excretion of phenyl acetate.

A.3. Laboratory investigations:

- Phenylalanine in blood: Normal level is 1 mg/dL. In PKU level increases >20 mg/dL.
- Ferric chloride test: Addition of ferric chloride in urine sample gives a transient blue-green color.
- Guthrie test—introduced by a microbiologist Guthrie, presence of high concentration of phenylalanine in blood overcome the effect of inhibitor on bacterial growth.
- Tandem mass spectroscopy—costly but most reliable.
- DNA probes

A.4. Early diagnosis plays important role, as approximate 5 units of IQ are lost for each 10 weeks delay in starting the treatment. For the first decade of life, child should be strictly on low phenylalanine (cassava diet). Sapropterin helps lower phenylalanine levels.

BIBLIOGRAPHY

1. Stone WL, Basit H, Los E. Phenylketonuria. [Updated 2022 Aug 8]. In: StatPearls [Internet]. Treasure Island (FL): StatPearls Publishing; 2022. Available from: https://www.ncbi.nlm.nih.gov/books/NBK535378/
2. Williams RA, Mamotte CD, Burnett JR. Phenylketonuria: an inborn error of phenylalanine metabolism. Clin Biochem Rev. 2008;29(1):31-41.

Case 2.6

Protein-Energy Malnutrition

COMPETENCY

❖ **BC8.3:** Describe the types and causes of protein energy malnutrition and its effects

Integration with Pediatrics

❖ **PE10.2:** Outline the clinical approach to a child with SAM and MAM

❖ **PE10.3:** Assessment of a patient with SAM and MAM, diagnosis, classification and planning management including hospital and community-based intervention, rehabilitation and prevention

Case Scenario

A 2-year-old child was brought to pediatric OPD with complains of watery diarrhea, edema of limbs, swelling over face and erythema of the skin. Child was lethargic and apathetic. Mother gave the history of weaning from last two months, usually with rice in diet. Laboratory tests were as follows.

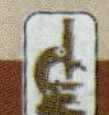

Laboratory Findings Reveal

- Hemoglobin—6.5 g% (12–16 g%)
- Total protein—3.8 g/dL (6–8 g/dL)
- Albumin—1.6 g/dL (3.5–5 g/dL)

QUESTIONS

Q.1. What is the probable diagnosis?

Q.2. Explain the biochemical basis of clinical finding in this patient.

Q.3. Enumerate the causes which leads to such clinical condition.

Q.4. How will you treat for protein-energy malnutrition?

ANSWERS

A.1. **Child is most probably suffering from malnutrition more specifically kwashiorkor. Kwashiorkor is a type of malnutrition characterized by severe protein deficiency. The characteristic features of kwashiorkor are hypoalbuminemia, poor wound healing and edema.**

A.2. Biochemical basis of sign and symptoms

Most of the signs and symptoms and clinical findings of kwashiorkor are due to low plasma protein and albumin levels. Functions of plasma proteins are:

- Immunity
- Blood clotting
- Maintaining blood pressure
- Maintaining blood volume
- Maintaining pH balance in the body

Decrease in plasma proteins leads to imbalance in all important functions, it reduces the osmotic pressure in blood vessels, result in edema. Decrease in plasma protein results in accumulation of VLDL/triglycerides in liver causes fatty liver. Clinical signs and symptoms are summarized in **Figure 2.6.1**.

- In preschool childern (1–5 years of age)
- Due to low protein intake
- Mild growth retardation
- Mild reduction in body weight
- Protruding abdomen and subcutaneous fat reserved
- Ribs not very prominent
- Poor appetite
- Enlarged fatty liver
- Edema present
- Moonfacies
- Sparse hair
- Flaky paint-like skin
- Lethargic
- Requies adequate amount of protein

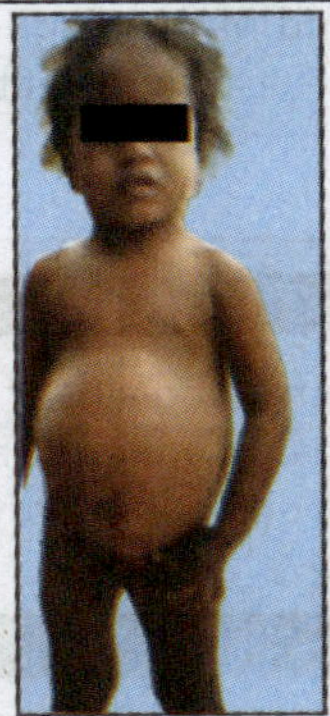

Kwashiorkor

- In weakened infants (<1 year old)
- Due to low calorie intake
- Severe growth retardation
- Severe reduction in bodyweight
- Shrunken abdomen and subcutaneous fat not preserved
- Prominent ribs
- Voracious feeder
- No fatty liver
- Edema not present
- An old man like face
- No hair changes noted
- Dry and wrinkled skin
- Alert but irritable
- Requires adequate amount of protein, fat and carbohydrate

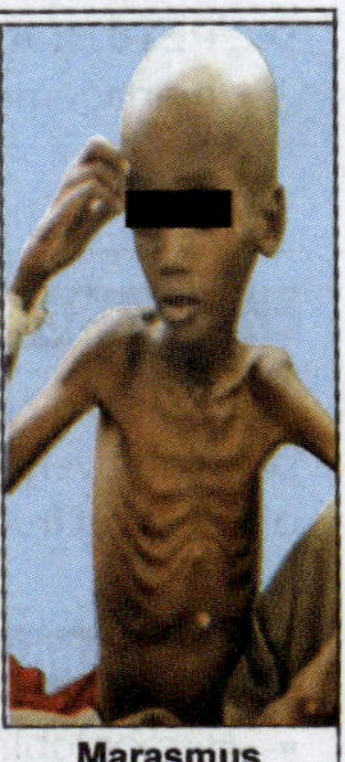

Marasmus

Fig. 2.6.1: Clinical presentation and difference between kwashiorkor and marasmus.

A.3. The primary causes associated with kwashiorkor are:

- Diet of mostly carbohydrates
- Weaning with inadequate food replacement.

Other factors that may contribute include:

- Lack of essential vitamins and minerals.
- Lack of dietary antioxidants.
- Aflatoxins—toxins from a mold that commonly grows on crops in hot and humid climates.
- Parasites and infectious diseases, particularly measles, malaria and HIV.

A.4. As per WHO guidelines following steps to follow to treat severe under nutrition:

One need to start cautious feeding and correct protein, micronutrient deficiencies as well electrolyte imbalances. Treatment/prevention is required for hypoglycemia, hypothermia, dehydration. Child needs sensory stimulation and emotional support. Regular follow-up should be done after recovery.

BIBLIOGRAPHY

1. https://apps.who.int/iris/bitstream/handle/10665/38925/9241541598_eng.pdf;jsessionid=B83F7A2E4C4EB97E99CA7BA9FD8E38B2?sequence=1
2. Mathew J, Sankar P, Varacallo M. Physiology, Blood Plasma. [Updated 2022 Apr 28]. In: StatPearls [Internet]. Treasure Island (FL): StatPearls Publishing; 2022. Available from: https://www.ncbi.nlm.nih.gov/books/NBK531504/

Case 2.7

Urea Cycle Disorders

COMPETENCY

❖ **BC5.6:** Describe the formation, transport, detoxification of Ammonia, Ammonia toxicity and its clinical significance

Integration with Medicine

❖ **GM5.5:** Describe and discuss the pathophysiology, clinical evolution and complications of cirrhosis of liver and portal hypertension including ascites, spontaneous bacterial peritonitis, hepato-renal syndrome, hepatic encephalopathy, acute GI bleed and hepatocellular carcinoma

Case Scenario

A 5-month-old female infant was admitted to hospital with a complaint of vomiting and a failure to gain weight. The mother also reported that the child would oscillate between periods of irritability and lethargy.

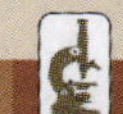

Laboratory Findings Reveal

Biochemical investigations of the patient

- Plasma ammonia—170 µg/dL (10–20 µg/dL)
- pH—7.55 (7.35–7.45)

QUESTIONS

Q.1. What is the most probable diagnosis? What can be the probable causes of the disorder?

Q.2. Explain the biochemical basis for the symptoms of this clinical condition.

Q.3. What will be the management for the patient?

ANSWERS

A.1. Child most probably suffering from urea cycle disorders which is a group of metabolic disorders resulting in hyperammonemia due to deficiency of one of the enzymes of urea cycle.

Causes of Hyperammonemia

Ammonia is the end product of protein metabolism and it is produced inside the cells of almost all tissues and reaches to liver for conversion into less toxic substance "urea". If due to some disease, toxins or inherited deficiency of enzymes, ammonia cannot be converted into urea, this will result in accumulation of ammonia leads to confusion and disorientation, excessive sleepiness, mood swings, hand tremors, coma and even death. Clinical signs and symptoms are summarized in **Figure 2.7.1.**

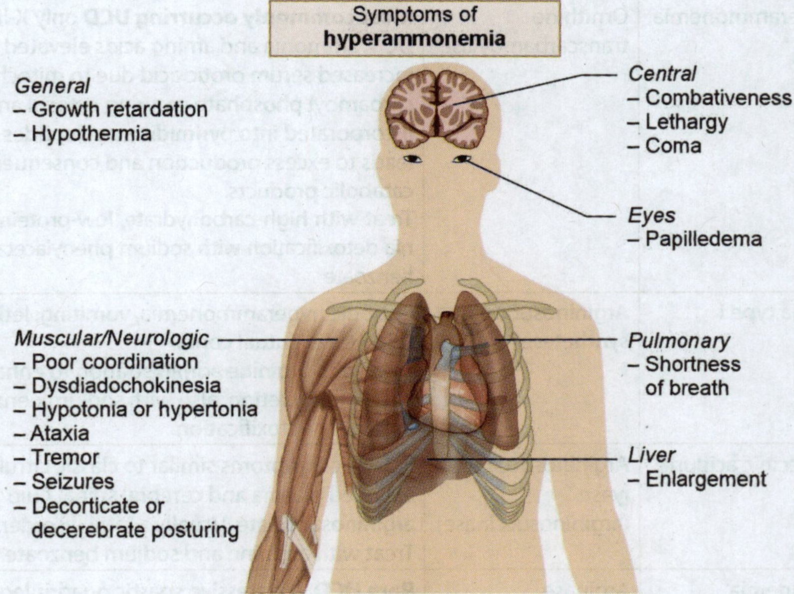

Fig. 2.7.1: Clinical presentation of hyperammonemia.

Types of Hyperammonemia

Acquired hyperammonemia: Acquired hyperammonemia is usually caused by diseases, toxins, hepatotoxic drugs that result in acute liver failure.

Inherited hyperammonemia: Inherited deficiency of urea cycle enzymes (details in **Table 2.7.1**).

Table 2.7.1: Classification of urea cycle disorders.

Urea cycle disorder (UCD)	*Enzyme deficiency*	*Symptoms/comments*
N-acetylglutamate synthetase deficiency	N-acetylglutamate synthetase	Severe to mild hyperammonemia, associated with deep coma, acidosis, recurrent diarrhea, ataxia, hypoglycemia, hyperornithinemia Treatment includes administration of carbamoyl glutamate to activate CPS-I

Contd...

Contd...

Urea cycle disorder (UCD)	*Enzyme deficiency*	*Symptoms/comments*
Type I hyperammonemia	Carbamoyl phosphate synthetase I	With 24-72h after birth infant becomes lethargic, needs stimulation to feed, vomiting, increasing lethargy, hypothermia, and hyperventilation; without measurement of serum ammonia levels and appropriate intervention infant will die. Treatment with arginine, which activates N-acetyl glutamate synthetase
Type 2 hyperammonemia	Ornithine transcarbamoylase	**Most commonly occurring UCD** only X-linked UCD, ammonia and amino acids elevated in serum, increased serum orotic acid due to mitochondrial carbamoyl phosphate entering cytosol and being incorporated into pyrimidine nucleotides which leads to excess production and consequently excess catabolic products. Treat with high-carbohydrate, low-protein diet, ammonia detoxification with sodium phenylacetate or sodium benzoate
Citrullinemia type I (CTLNI)	Argininosuccinate synthetase	Episodic hyperammonemia, vomiting, lethargy, ataxia, seizures, eventual coma. Treat with arginine administration to enhance citrulline excretion, also with sodium benzoate for ammonia detoxification
Argininosuccinic aciduria	Argininosuccinate lyase (argininosuccinase)	Episodic symptoms similar to classic citrullinemia, elevated plasma and cerebral spinal fluid argininosuccinate. Usually a fatal disorder. Treat with arginine and sodium benzoate
Hyperargininemia	Arginase	**Rare UCD**, progressive spastic quadriplegia and mental retardation; lysine, and arginine high in urine. Treatment includes diet of essential amino acids excluding arginine, low-protein diet

A.2. Biochemical basis for the symptoms of hyperammonemia are complex, possible explanation are:

a. **Direct toxic effect of ammonia on peripheral nerves**

b. **Ammonia has its toxic effect on brain: The brain tries to fix ammonia in the form of glutamine (it is the only amino acid can transport across the blood brain barrier) which results in increase level of glutamine in brain. Glutamine as osmotically active lead to neural cell swelling, neuronal damage and coma.**

c. **Glutamine synthesis is an energy requiring process and it utilizes glutamate as a precursor, which will result into:**

   1. **Depletion of GABA (an inhibitory neurotransmitter) which is synthesizes from glutamate.**
   2. **Depletion of α-ketoglutarate (one of the TCA cycle intermediate) as more of the α-ketoglutarate is diverted to form glutamate.**

A.3. Immediate treatment goal is a rapid lowering of ammonia, which can be achieve by:

- Reducing dietary protein intake
- Interrupt catabolic state by infusion of high calorie (carbohydrate + lipid)
- Remove excess ammonia by hemofiltration/hemodialysis which is very effective at reducing plasma ammonia
- Give arginine in order to support urea cycle
- Ammonia scavenger medications like sodium benzoate and phenylacetate (PA)/ phenylbutyrate (PB), modulate hepatic nitrogen metabolism mainly by providing alternative pathways for nitrogen disposal. Ammonia scavenger medications such as ammonul IV are also useful
- N-carbamylglutamate (Carbaglu) is an analogue of N-acetylglutamate, is found to be effective in NAGS deficiency and late-onset CPS1 deficiency
- Lactulose is also used to reduce the amount of ammonia in the blood of patients with liver disease
- In extreme cases liver transplantation is the choice of treatment.

BIBLIOGRAPHY

1. Ali R, Nagalli S. Hyperammonemia. [Updated 2022 Aug 8]. In: StatPearls [Internet]. Treasure Island (FL): StatPearls Publishing; 2022. Available from: https://www.ncbi.nlm.nih.gov/books/NBK557504/
2. Liu J, Lkhagva E, Chung HJ, Kim HJ, Hong ST. The Pharmabiotic Approach to Treat Hyperammonemia. Nutrients. 2018;10(2):140.

GIVE REASONS WHY

Q.1. Major transportation form of ammonia in blood is glutamic acid.

Ans. Most of the amino acids give their amino group to α ketoglutarate through transamination and forms glutamic acid. The concentration of glutamic acid in blood is approximately 10 times then the other amino acids. It can be significantly deaminate in the liver through glutamate dehydrogenase. However four amino acids directly deaminate their amino groups, e.g., lysine, threonine, proline and hydroxyproline. Glutamine is the transport form of ammonia from brain and intestine to liver, while alanine is the transport form from muscle.

Q.2. Negative nitrogen balance in fever.

Ans. Difference between nitrogen intake and excretion is known as nitrogen balance. A healthy human adult is in positive nitrogen balance. In fever and starvation, loss of nitrogen is greater than intake and the individual is in negative nitrogen balance.

Q.3. Proteolytic enzymes are secreted as zymogens.

Ans. Zymogens are inactive from of enzymes. They release inactive form to prevent auto-digestion of intestinal epithelium.

Q.4. Explain the egg allergy to some individuals.

Ans. In same individuals partially digested proteins particles directly absorb through para-cellularly (between epithelia cells) and enter in bloodstream. These partially digested protein particles act as an antigen and stimulate Ag-Ab type I hypersensitivity reaction.

Q.5. Chronic smoking leads to emphysema.

Ans. Enzyme α-1 antitrypsin prevents the breakdown of protein elastin, present in walls of alveoli of lungs. In chronic smokers the enzyme activity is decreased, causes breakdown of elastin leads to emphysema.

Q.6. Methylene is infused in treatment of methemoglobinemia.

Ans. Methylene blue keeps the iron in reduced form (ferrous from, Fe^{2+}). As in methemoglobinemia iron is oxidized (ferrous Fe^{2+} convert into ferric Fe^{3+}) form.

So, methylene blue is helpful in maintaining the iron in ferrous form and convert back the Fe^{3+} into Fe^{2+} form).

Q.7. Antihistamines are used to control allergic and anaphylactic reactions.

Ans. Antihistamines inhibits action of histamine. Histamine is an amine produce from decarboxylation of histidine. It is secreted from mast cells, basophils and platelets in response to certain allergens and causes antigen antibodies reaction, type I hypersensitive reactions. This is also known as anaphylaxis, characterized by vasodilation and fall in blood pressure.

Q.8. Melatonin can be useful for the workers having alternating day and night duties.

Ans. Melatonin is an acetylated serotonin (acetylated hydroxyl tryptamine) secreted from pineal gland. It is associated with regulation of diurnal variations, sleep awake cycles and biological rhythms. In small dose, it can induce sleep and can reset daily rhythm.

Q.9. Estimation of FIGLU in urine to diagnose/check folic acid deficiency.

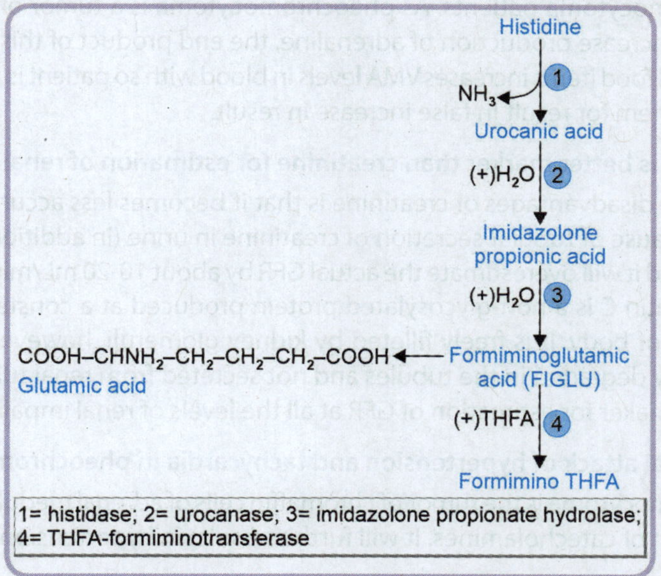

Ans. In histidine metabolism one the intermediate compound FIGLU (formiminoglutamic acid) is synthesized which gives its Formimino group to THFA (tetrahydrofolic acid) and results in formation of glutamic acid and forminimo THFA. Folic acid is essential for this metabolic reaction. Deficiency of folic acid increase serum level of FIGLU and its excretion in urine.

Q.10. Why there is burnt sweet smell in Maple syrup urine disease?

Ans. Maple syrup urine disease is a metabolic disorder of branched chain amino acids. There is deficiency of α keto acid dehydrogenase. Branched chain amino acids after transamination forms their respective keto acids, which cannot be further metabolized due to deficiency of above enzyme, it may result in accumulation of α keto acids which lead to burnt sweet small.

Q.11. Why thiamine is administered in Maple syrup urine disease?

Ans. In MSU disease usually enzyme α keto acid dehydrogenase in deficient. It is a complex enzyme which catalyzes oxidative decarboxylation and one of its coenzymes out of five coenzymes is thiamine.

Q.12. Carcinoid tumor causes deficiency of niacin.

Ans. Carcinoid tumor is a neuroendocrine tumor of small intestine, also known as "Argentaffinoma" which secretes large amounts of the serotonin. This neurotransmitter is synthesized from tryptophan and in this carcinoid condition excess of tryptophan is diverted to synthesize serotonin and very less is available to form niacin, causes deficiency of niacin.

Q.13. Chocolate, coffee, banana and vanilla, etc., restricted to pheochromocytoma patients.

Ans. Estimation of vanillylmandelic acid (VMA) in urine is one of the diagnostic test in pheochromocytoma patients. As pheochromocytoma is a tumor of adrenal medulla results in increase production of adrenaline, the end product of this is VMA, as above mentioned food items increases VMA levels in blood with so patient is advised to restrict intake of them for result in false increase in result.

Q.14. Cystatin C is better marker than creatinine for estimation of renal clearance.

Ans. One of the disadvantages of creatinine is that it becomes less accurate as GFR drops. This is because of tubular secretion of creatinine in urine (in addition to that which is filtered) and it will overestimate the actual GFR by about 10-20 mL/min. Where on other hand cystatin C is a non-glycosylated protein produced at a constant rate in almost all organs of body. It is freely filleted by kidney glomeruli, however reabsorbed but completely degraded in the tubules and not secreted from renal tubules makes it an excellent maker for estimation of GFR at all the levels of renal impairment.

Q.15. Paroxysmal attack of hypertension and tachycardia in pheochromocytoma.

Ans. Pheochromocytoma is the tumor of chromaffin cells of adrenal medulla, leads to excess production of catecholamines. It will further results in hypertension and tachycardia.

Q.16. Hypoalbuminemia results in tissue edema.

Ans. Proteins in blood is to provide EOP (effective oncotic pressure) and prevent the movement of water from blood vessels to the extracellular space. If the level of protein reduces in blood vessels, it will result in release of water from blood vessels to the extra vascular space resulting in edema. It is seen when albumin level in blood is less than 2 g/dL and this occurs in following condition:

- Malnutrition—generalized edema.
- Nephrotic syndrome—generalized edema.
- Cirrhosis—ascites fluid in peritoneal cavity.
- Chronic congestive cardiac failure—generalized edema.

Q.17. Aspartame should be avoided as artificial sweetener in phenylketonuria.

Ans. Aspartame is consisting of aspartic acid and phenylalanine dipeptide. As the use of the sweetener increases phenylalanine concentration. It should be avoided in phenylketonuria.

Q.18. Estimation of xanthurenic acid in urine to detect PLP deficiency.

Ans. PLP is required as a coenzyme in tryptophan metabolism during conversion of kynurenine into hydroxyanthranilic acid. In the PLP deficiency kynurenine levels increases and diverts to from xanthurenic acid. Excess of xanthurenic acid in urine indicates PLP deficiency.

Section 3

Lipid Metabolism

- ❖ **Case 3.1:** Chyluria
- ❖ **Case 3.2:** Fatty Liver
- ❖ **Case 3.3:** Hypertriglyceridemia with Acute Pancreatitis
- ❖ **Case 3.4:** Niemann-Pick Disease
- ❖ **Case 3.5:** Phrynoderma
- ❖ **Case 3.6:** Refsum Disease
- ❖ **Case 3.7:** Respiratory Distress Syndrome
- ❖ **Case 3.8:** Zellweger Syndrome

Give Reasons Why

Case 3.1

Chyluria

COMPETENCY

- **BC4.2:** Describe the digestion and absorption of dietary lipids and its associated disorders
- **BC4.4:** Describe metabolism of Triglycerides and cholesterol metabolism along with its regulation and clinical significance

Case Scenario

A 45-year-old thin built woman presented with complaints of milky white urination for the last 8 years. There was report of weakness, loss of weight, mild pain in the flanks and psychologically upset for a long time illness. The patient was a resident an endemic zone of lymphatic filariasis. The patient consulted one gynecologist for treatment of white discharge which mimics chyluria.

On microscopical examination of the sediment of the urine, *Candida albicans* and *Trichomonas vaginalis* were not detected. Ultrasonography of the abdomen did not reveal any pathology. The patient was suffering from type-2 diabetes and undergoing treatment by an endocrinologist with oral hypoglycemic drugs. The patient was taking Glimepiride (1 mg) + Metformin (500 mg) twice daily before food and one tablet Metformin (1000 mg) before dinner.

The sugar level was not under control, blood HbA1c level is 8.5%, high serum triglyceride (196 mg/dL), serum protein (6.8 g/dL) and serum albumin (3.7 g/dL) were found to be within reference value. The urine examination revealed the presence of protein, sugar (0.5%) and chyle in very high quantity, without red blood cells.

QUESTIONS

Q.1. What is the probable diagnosis? Explain biochemical basis of such clinical condition.

Q.2. What are the diagnostic modalities available to confirm your diagnosis?

Q.3. What are the factors required to transport lipids in the blood? Write the significance of phospholipids in these complexes.

Q.4. What is the management in such clinical condition?

ANSWERS

A.1. This is a case of chyluria. Majority of the absorbed lipids such as triacylglycerols, phospholipids, cholesterol, cholesterol ester and fat soluble vitamins forms chylomicrons that form a milky fluid, the chyle. The size of this lipid complex makes it unable to pass through endothelial cells of the capillaries (without prior hydrolysis). That is why, it is collected by the lymphatic vessels of the abdominal region and further in systemic circulation via the thoracic duct. If any abnormal connection is formed between the urinary tract and the lymphatic drainage system of the intestine, known as chylous fistula, it will result in excretion of lipid complex chylomicrons in the urine.

The similar abnormality, chylothorax is found when the abnormal connection is formed between pleural space and lymphatic vessels of the abdominal region.

A.2. Diagnosis of chyluria or chylous urine can be done by following process:

- **Examination of chyluria or chylous urine:** Milky appearance of the urine contains gel, blood and fibrin clots. Examination of urine after sometime indicates separation of layers. Top layer consist of fat, middle layer contains fibrin and bottom layer contains cells and debris **(Fig. 3.1.1)**.

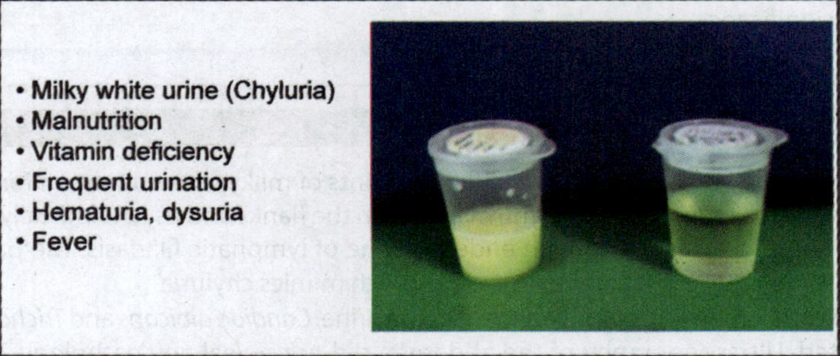

Fig. 3.1.1: Clinical presentation of chyluria.

- **Lab investigations to diagnose chyluria or chylous urine**
  - *Ether test:* Chyluria when mixed with ether the opacity disappears.
  - *Methylene blue test:* Test shows presence of lymphocytes.
  - *Sudan III test:* Sudan III indicator is ingested with fatty food. Urine sample is collected after 2 to 6 hours. Urine color is orange-pink.
  - *Immunoelectrophoresis for Chyluria or Chylous Urine:* Immunoelectrophoresis shows globulins of intestinal origin (Apo B-48).
  - *Cystourethroscopy for chyluria or chylous urine:* Cystoscopy and urethroscopy is performed to evaluate the source of chyles in urine.
- **Radiological studies for chyluria or chylous urine**
  - Intravenous pyelography
  - CT scans of kidney, ureter, bladder and urethra.
  - MRI scan: Kidney, ureter and bladder
  - Ultrasonography
  - Lymphangiography
  - Lymphangioscintigraphy
  - Renal biopsy

A.3. Proteins, phospholipids and cholesterol are responsible for the transport of lipoprotein complexes in the circulation. Phospholipids help in movement of lipoproteins in circulation as well due to presence of unsaturated fatty acids in its structure it helps in reverse cholesterol transport (bring the cholesterol back from extrahepatic to the liver, and reduces the cholesterol level in blood).

A.4. Patient should be advised to take short or medium chain fatty acids in lipid diet, as these fatty acids are directly absorbed through intestine and enter in hepatic portal circulation rather than as chylomicrons in the thoracic duct.

Anti-filarial drug: Diethylcarbamazine can be used for filariasis. Sclerotherapy and surgery are the last option when all conservative treatment fails.

BIBLIOGRAPHY

1. Dalela D. Issues in etiology and diagnosis making of chyluria. Indian J Urol. 2005;21:18-23.
2. Stainer V, Jones P, Juliebø SØ, Beck R, Hawary A. Chyluria: What does the clinician need to know? Ther Adv Urol. 2020;12:1756287220940899.

Case 3.2

Fatty Liver

COMPETENCY

- ❖ **BC4.7:** Describe Fatty liver, cholelithiasis and obesity
- ❖ **BC4.8:** Interpret laboratory results of analytes associated with metabolism of lipids
- ❖ **BC13.4:** Discuss metabolism of alcohol with biochemical changes and effects of chronic alcoholism

Case Scenario

A 55-year-old executive male with past medical history of borderline diabetes presents to you with abnormal liver enzymes discovered 6 months ago. History of alcohol consumption and smoking for last 10 years, family history revels that his mother died from end-stage liver disease few years back. On physical examination mild hepatomegaly was there.

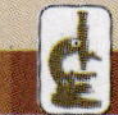

Laboratory Findings Reveal

- Serum AST—176 IU/L (8–20 IU/L)
- Serum ALT—148 IU/L (10–40 IU/L)
- Serum total protein—4.5 g/dL (6–8 g/dL)
- Serum albumin—2 g/L (3.5–5 g/dL)

Liver ultrasonography showed diffuse increase in echogenicity and vascular blurring consistent with fatty infiltration.

QUESTIONS

Q.1. What is the most probable diagnosis of this clinical condition?

Q.2. What is the biochemical basis for the above condition?

Q.3. How chronic alcoholism predisposes this clinical condition?

Q.4. How you confirm your diagnosis?

Q.5. How lipotropic factors prevent fatty liver?

ANSWERS

A.1. Patients most probably suffering from fatty liver. Clinical signs and symptoms are summarized in **Figure 3.2.1**.

Fatty liver is also known as hepatic steatosis. Normally small amount of fat is present in liver, but fatty liver is a pathologic condition, where extensive accumulation of fat (triacylglycerol) occurs in hepatocytes (more than 10% of liver weight). Fatty liver can be classified as:

- Alcoholic fatty liver disease, also called alcoholic steatohepatitis
- Non-alcoholic fatty liver disease (NAFLD), also called non-alcoholic steatohepatitis (NASH). This is the common hepatic disorder.

Another clinical condition which occurs during pregnancy known as (k/a) acute fatty liver of pregnancy (AFLP), which is a rare but serious pregnancy complication.

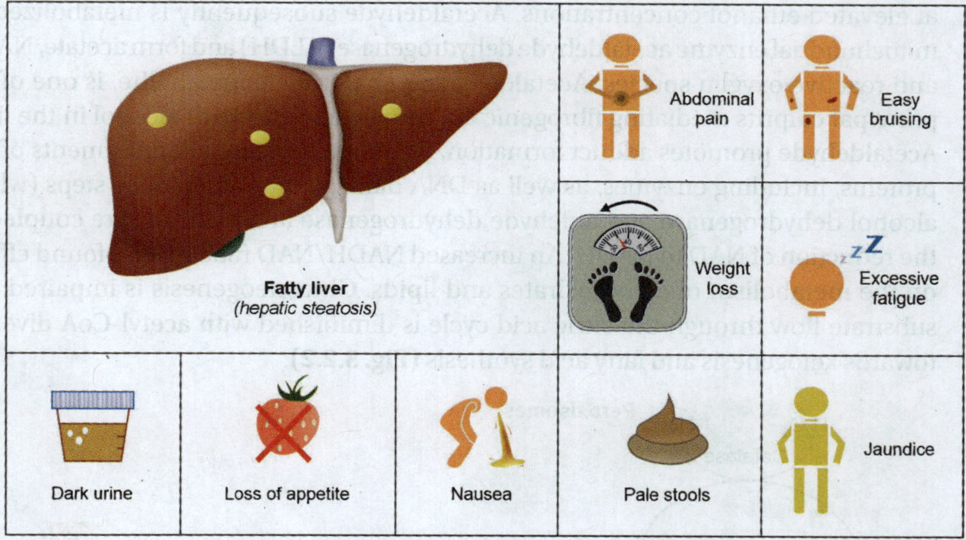

Fig. 3.2.1: Clinical presentation of fatty liver.

A.2. Biochemical Basis of Fatty Liver

Metabolic disturbance in fatty liver results in:

- Raised level of plasma free fatty acids: Increase mobilization of fatty acids from adipose tissue (increase in hormone sensitive lipase) to the liver for example in uncontrolled diabetes, starvation, feeding high fat diets. This increase influx of fatty acids in liver results in excess formation, and accumulation of triglycerides in the liver.
- Block in the transport of lipoproteins from liver to blood. Deficiency of two important factors protein and phospholipids require for the movement of lipoproteins from liver to circulation may cause accumulation of lipoproteins in hepatocytes. When accumulation of lipid in the liver becomes chronic, fibrotic changes occur in the hepatic cells that progress to cirrhosis and impaired liver functions.

A.3. Fatty Liver in Alcoholism

Within the liver, main enzymes involved in alcohol metabolism:

- Alcohol dehydrogenase mechanism
- Cytochrome P-450 2E1 (CYP2E1)
- Catalase
- Aldehyde dehydrogenase

Alcohol dehydrogenase (ADH) is a hepatocyte cytosolic enzyme that converts alcohol to acetaldehyde. Catalase, located in cell bodies called peroxisomes, requires hydrogen peroxide (H_2O_2) to oxidize alcohol. CYP2E1, present predominantly in the cell's microsomes, assumes an important role in metabolizing ethanol to acetaldehyde at elevated ethanol concentrations. Acetaldehyde subsequently is metabolized by mitochondrial enzyme acetaldehyde dehydrogenase (ALDH) and form acetate, NADH and reactive oxygen species. Acetaldehyde, a major toxic metabolite, is one of the principal culprits mediating fibrogenic and mutagenic effects of alcohol in the liver. Acetaldehyde promotes adduct formation, leading to functional impairments of key proteins, including enzymes, as well as DNA damage. Both metabolic steps (where alcohol dehydrogenase and aldehyde dehydrogenase are involved) are coupled to the reduction of NAD to NADH. An increased NADH/NAD ratio has profound effects on the metabolism of carbohydrates and lipids. Gluconeogenesis is impaired and substrate flow through the citric acid cycle is diminished with acetyl-CoA diverted towards ketogenesis and fatty acid synthesis **(Fig. 3.2.2)**.

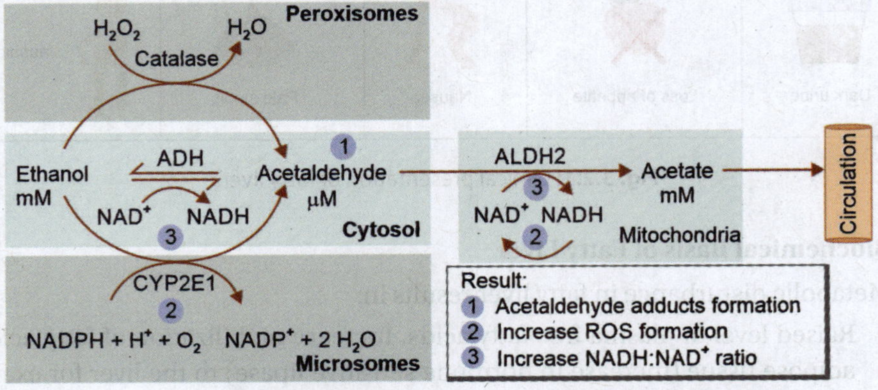

Fig. 3.2.2: Alcohol metabolism.

A.4. With combination of biochemical investigation, radiological imaging and liver biopsy diagnosis of fatty can be confirmed.

- **Biochemistry evaluation**
  Liver function tests: Increased levels of the liver enzymes alanine aminotransferase (ALT) and aspartate aminotransferase (AST)
- **Radiological imaging**
  Abdominal ultrasound, computerized tomography (CT) scanning or magnetic resonance imaging (MRI) of the abdomen.

Elastography: It is a newer type of imaging test that measure the stiffness of liver tissue. Increased liver stiffness may be a sign of fibrosis.

- **Liver biopsy:** This is the only confirmatory diagnostic test which can predict the severity of disease earlier than imaging technique but due to its invasive nature this is last choice of investigation, when other is inconclusive.

A.5. Lipotropic Factors

Substances that hasten the removal or decrease the deposition of fat in the liver through their interaction with fat metabolism known as lipotropic factors.

- Molecules require to synthesize phospholipids like choline, ethanolamine, inositol serine, essential fatty acid, etc.
- Antioxidant vitamins and mineral—vitamin-C, E and A, selenium—antioxidant vitamins and minerals prevent the oxidation of PUFA used in formation of phospholipids.
- Others—betaine hydrochloride, oxibetaine.

BIBLIOGRAPHY

1. Horn P, Newsome PN. Nonalcoholic Fatty Liver Disease. N Engl J Med. 2022;386(3):294.
2. Mir BA, Majeed T, Chauhan A. Nonalcoholic Fatty Liver Disease. N Engl J Med. 2022;386(3):295.
3. Stengel JZ, Harrison SA. Nonalcoholic Steatohepatitis: Clinical Presentation, Diagnosis, and Treatment. Gastroenterol Hepatol (NY). 2006;2(6):440-449.

Case 3.3

Hypertriglyceridemia with Acute Pancreatitis

COMPETENCY

- ❖ **BC4.4:** Describe metabolism of Triglycerides and cholesterol metabolism along with its regulation and clinical significance
- ❖ **BC14.19:** Explain the basis and rationale of biochemical tests done and interpretation of laboratory results in Pancreatitis

Case Scenario

A 46-year-old man was referred from the accident and emergency (A&E) department with 7 days of abdominal pain and yellow pustular skin eruptions on his arms and torso. His abdominal pain was worse after eating, and was associated with nausea. He denied any diarrhea or vomiting and had no urinary symptoms.

On examination: Physical examination revealed a fever of 38.5°F, tachycardia of 100, blood pressure of 120/70 mm Hg, respiratory rate of 16 and saturating 95% on air. He had abdominal tenderness in his right upper quadrant.

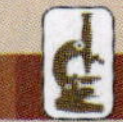

Laboratory Findings Reveal

Serum after centrifugation was milky in color (lipemic):

- Serum lipid profile
- Total cholesterol: 210 mg/dL (normal up to 200 mg/dL)
- LDL cholesterol: 108 mg/dL (normal <100 mg/dL)
- HDL cholesterol: 30 mg/dL (normal >40 mg/dL)
- Serum triglyceride: 360 mg/dL (normal <150 mg/dL)
- VLDL cholesterol: 72 mg/dL (normal <40 mg/dL)
- Serum lipase: 480 IU/L (normal 0–160 IU/L)
- Serum amylase: 760 IU/L (normal 40–140 IU/L)
- Blood sugar: 168 mg/dL (normal random sugar—70–140 mg/dL)
- Blood pH: 7.0 (normal 7.35–7.45)

QUESTIONS

Q.1. What is the most probable diagnosis of this patient? Enumerate causative agents of this clinical condition.

Q.2. How you confirm your diagnosis?

Q.3. What is the line of management?

ANSWERS

A.1. Patient is most probably suffering from acute pancreatitis which could be due to viral or bacterial infection (high grade fever). Clinical signs and symptoms of acute pancreatitis are summarized in **Figure 3.3.1**. Other clinical conditions which can leads to acute pancreatitis are:

- Moderate or severe alcohol consumption
- Gallbladder stones
- Obesity
- Certain medication
- Hormonal abnormality.

There are some general symptoms that may indicate acute/chronic pancreatitis, include:

- Severe abdominal pain having food
- Pain in upper abdominal pain that goes back
- Rapid heart beat
- Upset stomach
- Fever
- Unwanted weight loss
- Nausea and vomiting
- Stinking and oily stool
- Tender and swollen belly
- Diarrhea
- Bleeding
- Dehydraion

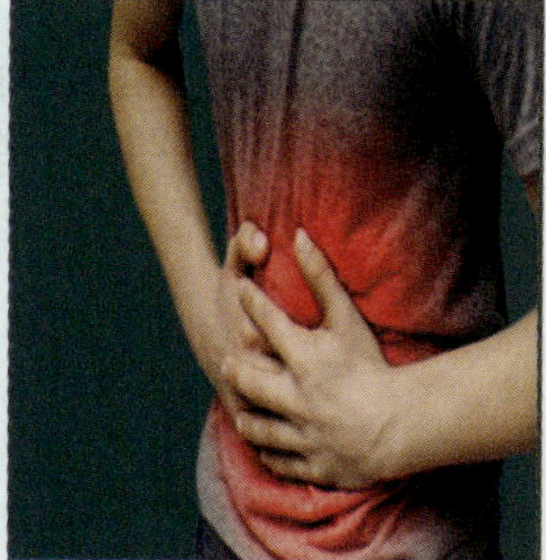

Fig. 3.3.1: Clinical presentation of pancreatitis.

A.2. Investigations for confirmation of acute pancreatitis are as follows:

- Serum lipase: It raises late but more specific compare to serum amylase which is sensitive but less specific.
- Abdominal ultrasonography: Ultrasonography of the abdomen is the most useful initial test in determining the etiology of pancreatitis and is the technique of choice for detecting gallstones. In the setting of acute pancreatitis, sensitivity remain up to 70–80%.
- Magnetic resonance cholangiopancreatography (MRCP): MRCP uses magnetic resonance imaging, a non-invasive test that produces cross-section images of parts of the body.
- Computerized tomography (CT) scan

Other supportive investigations which can be helpful are:

- Total blood count
- Liver function test

Box 3.1 depicts the diagnostic criteria of acute pancreatitis.

Box 3.1: Diagnostic criteria of acute pancreatitis.
1. Typical abdominal pain
2. Three or more times elevation of pancreatic enzymes
3. Inflammation of the gland on CT or MRI

A.3. Management of acute pancreatitis include:

- Intravenous fluid to treat dehydration, nil by mouth for few days.
- Analgesics and antibiotics through an intravenous line or by mouth if possible.
- A low-fat diet or nutrition by feeding tube or intravenous.

BIBLIOGRAPHY

1. Chatila AT, Bilal M, Guturu P. Evaluation and management of acute pancreatitis. World J Clin Cases. 2019;7(9):1006-1020.
2. Gapp J, Chandra S. Acute Pancreatitis. [Updated 2022 Jun 21]. In: StatPearls [Internet]. Treasure Island (FL): StatPearls Publishing; 2022. Available from: https://www.ncbi.nlm.nih.gov/books/NBK482468/

Case 3.4

Niemann-Pick Disease

COMPETENCY

❖ **BC4.8:** Interpret laboratory results of analytes associated with metabolism of Lipids

Case Scenario

A 4-year-old boy brought to OPD by his mother with complain of failure to grow and distension of abdomen. There was also history of intermittent fever, difficulty in walking in the form of repeated falls and multiple episodes of tonic-clonic seizures since last 1 year. Careful examination reveals hepatosplenomegaly, neurodevelopmental delay. Bone marrow biopsy reveals lipid laden histiocyte, known as foamy cells. Fundoscopy shows macular cherry red spots.

QUESTIONS

Q.1. What is the most probable diagnosis of this clinical condition?

Q.2. How will you explain the biochemical basis for the same?

Q.3. How you confirm your diagnosis? Enlist the three disorders in the differential diagnosis of this clinical condition.

Q.4. What is the line of management?

ANSWERS

A.1. Child is most probably suffering from Niemann-Pick disease. This is an autosomal recessive disorder which is one of inherited metabolic disorders known as lipid storage diseases that affect the body's ability to metabolize fat (cholesterol and lipids) within cells. Clinical signs and symptoms are summarized in **Figure 3.4.1**.

A.2. Niemann-Pick disease is characterized by absence of sphingomyelinase results in accumulation of sphingomyelin in various tissues like in the brain, spleen, liver, skin and lung resulting in clinical presentation of disease.

A.3. The diagnose can be achieved by quantitative analysis of sphingomyelin in the liver, spleen, leukocytes and kidney, or measuring the acid sphingomyelinase activity level in peripheral leukocytes or cultured fibroblasts. Prenatal diagnosis can be made by measuring the acid sphingomyelinase activity level in cultured amniocytes or chorionic villi.

Types and presentation

Type A: Infancy
Skin: Xanthomas; yellow brown, waxy induration on exposed surfaces
Central nervous system: Progressive psychomotor deterioration, hypotonicity, muscle weakness
Gastrointestinal: Hepatosplenomegaly, emaciated appearance failure to thrive, vomiting
Lymphatics: Generalized enlarged lymph nodes
Eyes: Blindness, cherry red spots
Ear, nose, throat: Deafness
Lungs: Bronchopneumonia, infiltration of foam cells

Type B: Infancy to childhood
CNS spared, otherwise similar to type A

Type C: Childhood
Developmental delay, hepatosplenomegaly, progressive psychomotor deterioration

Signs and symptoms of Niemann-Pick disease

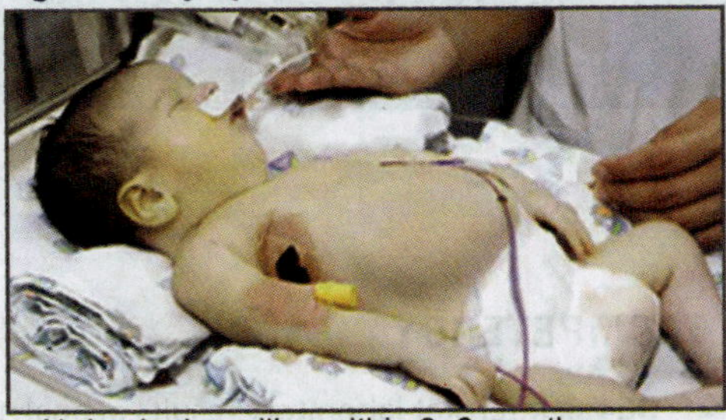

- Abdominal swelling within 3–6 months
- Loss of appetite
- Loss of early motor skills
- Enlarged spleen and liver
- Jaundice at birth
- Irregular speech

Fig. 3.4.1: Clinical presentation of Niemann-Pick disease.

A.4. Currently, there is no specific treatment for Niemann-Pick disease. Splenectomy, bone marrow transplantation, liver transplantation and amniotic cell transplantation have been attempted but had little or no success.

Cyclodextrin and histone deacetylase inhibitors are found to be effective in slowing progression of Niemann-Pick disease.

BIBLIOGRAPHY

1. Bajwa H, Azhar W. Niemann-Pick Disease. [Updated 2022]. In: StatPearls [Internet]. Treasure Island (FL): StatPearls Publishing; 2022. Available from: https://www.ncbi.nlm.nih.gov/books/NBK556129.
2. https://www.ninds.nih.gov/health-information/disorders/niemann-pick-disease.

Case 3.5

Phrynoderma

COMPETENCY

- **BC4.1:** Describe and discuss main classes of lipids and their functions
- **BC4.6:** Discuss Biological role and therapeutic applications of Eicosanoids and their Inhibitors

Case Scenario

A 24-year-old woman who had put on weight after childbirth was advised by her physician to reduce her calorie intake. Being impatient she stopped consuming fats and oils . Though she lost the excess weight, after a few months, she developed skin lesions on limbs and arms.

QUESTIONS

Q.1. Identify the case. Explain the biochemical basis for above condition.

Q.2. What are essential fatty acids? Enumerate them.

Q.3. What role do eicosanoids play in the body?

ANSWERS

A.1. Patient most probably suffering from phrynoderma. It is a distinctive form of follicular hyperkeratosis **associated with nutritional deficiency** due to deficiency of vitamin A and essential fatty acids. Clinical signs and symptoms are summarized in **Figure 3.5.1**.

- Follicular hyperkeratosis
- Cheilitis, glossitis
- Blepharitis
- Diarrhea
- Muscle weakness
- Neuritis

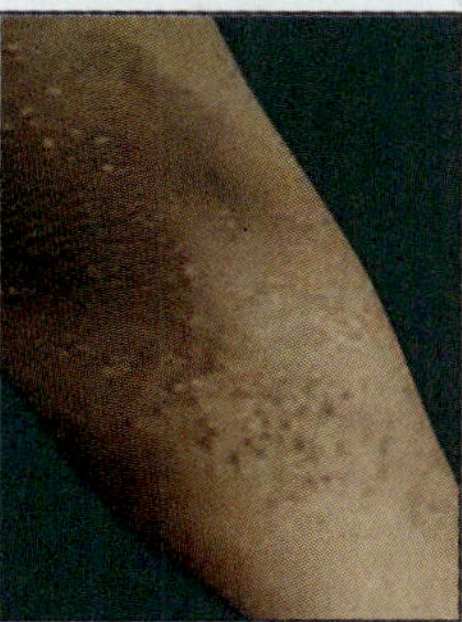

Fig. 3.5.1: Clinical presentation of phrynoderma.

A.2. Essential fatty acids: Those fatty acids which are essential for growth and development but humans cannot synthesize them.

- Linoleic acid
- Alpha linolenic acids
- Arachidonic acids.

Arachidonic acid can be synthesized from linoleic acid, so arachidonic acid also known as semi-essential fatty acid.

A.3. Arachidonic acid is an essential fatty acid and a precursor in the biosynthesis of prostaglandins, thromboxane, and leukotriene's **(Fig. 3.5.2)**.

Thromboxane are synthesized in platelets and upon release cause vasoconstriction and platelet aggregation.

Prostacyclins (PGI2) are potent inhibitors of platelet aggregation.

Leukotrienes are constrictor of the bronchial airway musculature.

Lipoxins are vasoactive and have immunoregulatory functions.

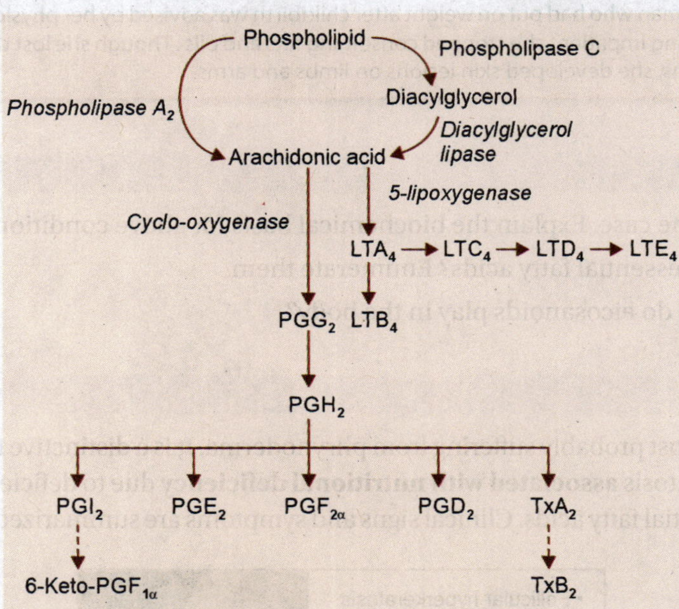

Fig. 3.5.2: Synthesis of prostaglandins.

BIBLIOGRAPHY

1. Chia MW, Tay YK, Liu TT. Phrynoderma: a forgotten entity in a developed country. Singapore Med J. 2008;49(6):e160-2.
2. Heath ML, Sidbury R. Cutaneous manifestations of nutritional deficiency. Curr Opin Pediatr. 2006;18(4):417-22.

Case 3.6

Refsum Disease

COMPETENCY

❖ **BC4.8:** Interpret laboratory results of analytes associated with metabolism of Lipids

Case Scenario

A 2-year 9-month-old girl with nystagmus, visual and hearing impairment, and developmental delay admitted in pediatric ward. Her medical history was otherwise unremarkable with a normal pregnancy and delivery. There was no history of genetic disorders in the family. On examination child had motor unsteadiness and frequent nosebleeds. For last six months child deteriorated neurologically with increased swallowing difficulty, choking and gagging during eating. She also had increasing difficulty with walking, along with increased nystagmus.

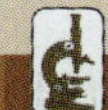

Laboratory Findings Reveal

Elevation of very long chain fatty acids in serum.

QUESTIONS

Q.1. What is the most probable diagnosis?

Q.2. What are the biochemical basis of your diagnosis?

Q.3. How you confirm your diagnosis?

Q.4. What is the line of management?

ANSWERS

A.1. Child most probably suffering from Refsum disease. This metabolic disorder inherited as an autosomal recessive manner. Clinical sign and symptoms are summarized in **Figure 3.6.1**.

A.2. Biochemical basis of refsum disease. The lack of function of the enzyme (phytanoyl-CoA hydroxylase) leads to a build-up of phytanic acid in blood plasma and tissues. Phytanic acid accumulates in our nerve, liver and fat tissues which leads to the dysfunction of the myelin in the central and peripheral nervous systems.

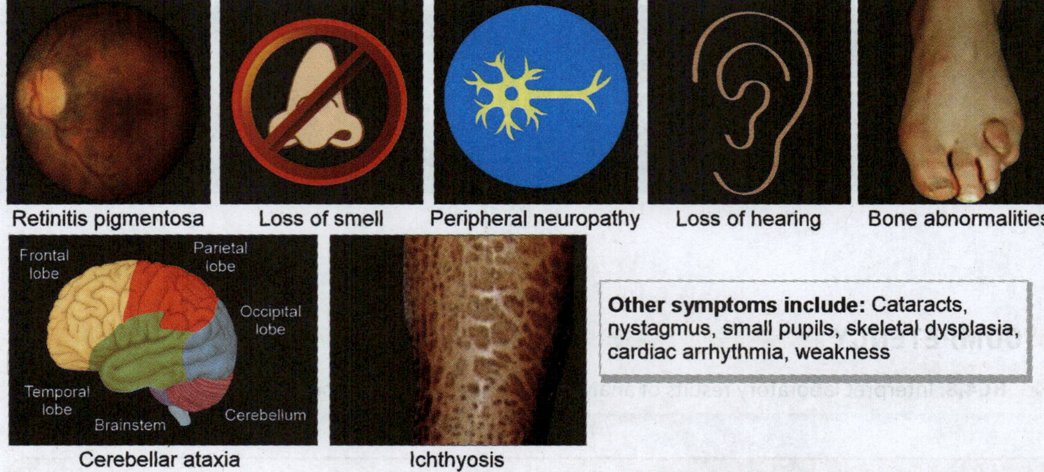

Fig. 3.6.1: Clinical presentation of refsum disease.

A.3. Refsum disease can be diagnosed by:
- Blood test for elevated levels of phytanic acid—10 to 50 mg/dL (normal level ≥0.2 mg/dL)
- *Genetic testing:* Mutation in PHYH gene (≈ 90%) or mutation in PEX7 gene.
- *Fibroblast test:* Defect in phytanic oxidase activity in fibroblast.

A.4. Current treatment strategies include maintenance of low phytanic acid levels in blood and symptomatic care of patients this includes:
- Low phytanic acid diet: Either by dietary restrictions and/or plasmapheresis or lipid apheresis
- Symptomatic management include cataract surgery, eye drops, hearing aids, cochlear implants, skin lotions, pain management.

BIBLIOGRAPHY

1. Kumar R, De Jesus O. Refsum Disease. [Updated 2022]. In: StatPearls [Internet]. Treasure Island (FL): StatPearls Publishing; 2022. Available from: https://www.ncbi.nlm.nih.gov/books/NBK560618.
2. Wierzbicki AS, Lloyd MD, Schofield CJ, Feher MD, Gibberd FB. Refsum's disease: a peroxisomal disorder affecting phytanic acid alpha-oxidation. J Neurochem. 2002;80(5):727-35.

Case 3.7

Respiratory Distress Syndrome

COMPETENCY

- ❖ **BC4.1:** Describe and discuss main classes of lipids and their functions

Integration with Pediatrics

- ❖ **PE19.5:** Describe the etiology, clinical features and management of Respiratory distress in Newborn including meconium aspiration and transient tachypnea of newborn

Case Scenario

A newborn which was delivered premature, presenting with difficulty in breathing, increased respiratory rate, cyanosis, tachypnea (RR >70/min), nasal flaring and poor feeding. His condition was progressively worsening and he was put on oxygen. X-ray chest finding reveals ground glass appearance.

QUESTIONS

Q.1. What is the most probable diagnosis? Explain biochemical basis of this clinical condition.

Q.2. How you confirm your diagnosis? Whether it can be diagnosed in antenatal period.

Q.3. What is neonatal hyaline membrane disease?

Q.4. What is the management of this clinical condition?

ANSWERS

A.1. Neonate is most probably suffering from respiratory distress syndrome. Clinical signs and symptoms are summarized in **Figure 3.7.1**.

It usually develops within the first 6–24 hours after birth, symptoms include rapid, shallow breathing and a sharp, pulling-in of the chest below and between the ribs with each breath **(Fig. 3.7.2)**.

Biochemical Basis of Disease

This clinical condition occurs due to impaired synthesis of pulmonary surfactant, which is found at the air water interface of alveoli. Pulmonary surfactant reduces the

- Severe shortness of breath
- Labored and unusually rapid breathing/ fast and shallow breathing
- Grunting, low blood pressure
- Flaring of the nostrils with each breath
- Cyanosis
- Indrawing of lower chest

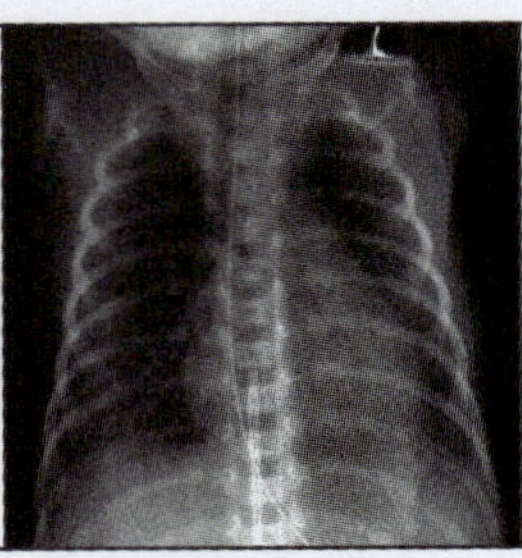

Fig. 3.7.1: Clinical presentation of respiratory distress syndrome.

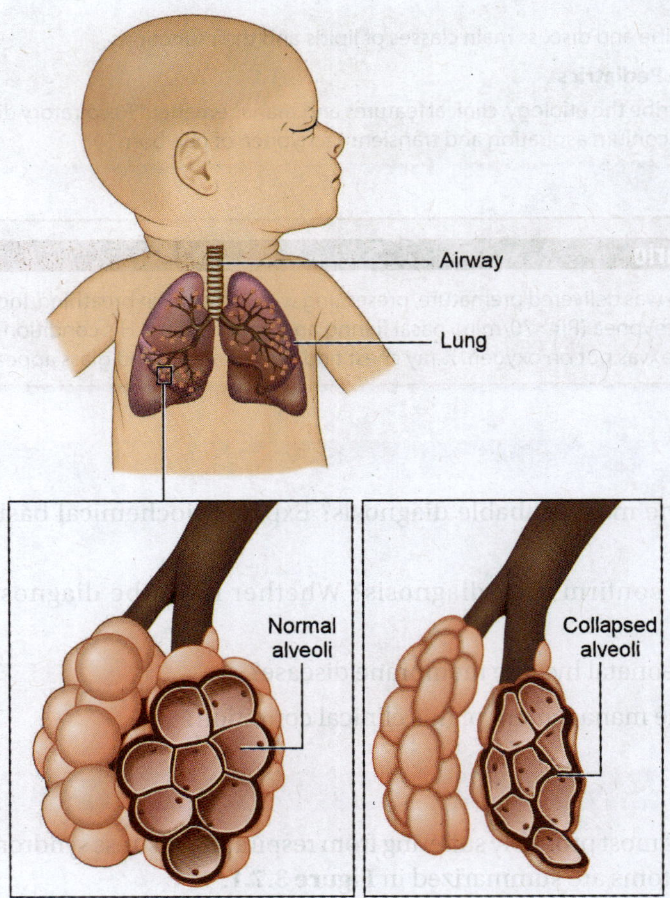

Fig. 3.7.2: Diagrammatic representations of alveoli in respiratory distress syndrome.

surface tension at the air-liquid interface of the alveoli, thus preventing its collapse during end exhalation.

Pulmonary surfactant is a surface-active complex of phospholipids and proteins formed by type II alveolar cells. Its composition is mentioned in **Table 3.7.1**.

Table 3.7.1: Composition of pulmonary surfactant.		
Phospholipids: 70–80%	***Proteins: 10%***	***Others: 10%***
Lecithin (phosphatidylcholine) Dipalmitoylphosphatidylcholine (DCPP) also k/a dipalmitoyl lecithin **(strongest surfactant)**	Surfactant protein (A, B, C and D)	Cholesterol

A.2. Diagnosis can be made by:

- Typical ground glass appearance on X-ray chest
- Antenatal diagnosis: For antenatal diagnosis of lung maturity estimation of lecithin/sphingomyelin (L/S) ratio is done in amniotic fluid. Ratio more than 2:1 indicates lung maturity.

A.3. Neonatal hyaline membrane disease, also known as neonatal respiratory distress syndrome. It results due to insufficient production of respiratory surfactant mainly the surfactant proteins. There is the appearance of waxy, hyaline membrane lining the alveoli of lung. It is composed of cellular debris, blood cells and fibrin, this makes the alveoli unable for the exchange of gases across the alveolar membrane.

A.4. Treatment Consists of Supportive Care

Treatment includes medication to keep the lungs open, breathing support and oxygen therapy.

Oxygen Supplement

Nasal cannula

For milder symptoms or as a temporary measure, oxygen may be delivered through a mask.

Mechanical ventilation

Most people with ARDS need the help of a machine to breathe.

Continuous positive airway pressure (CPAP): This machine gently pushes air or oxygen into the lungs to keep the air sacs open.

Ventilator (for severe RDS): This is a machine that helps the infant breathe when they cannot breathe well enough without help.

Pharmacological Support—Surfactant Therapy

Methylprednisolone (Solu-Medrol): High-dose methylprednisolone has been used in trials of patients with ARDS who have persistent pulmonary infiltrates, fever, and high oxygen requirement.

BIBLIOGRAPHY

1. Diamond M, Peniston HL, Sanghavi D, et al. Acute Respiratory Distress Syndrome. [Updated 2022 Sep 21]. In: StatPearls [Internet]. Treasure Island (FL): StatPearls Publishing; 2022. Available from: https://www.ncbi.nlm.nih.gov/books/NBK436002.
2. https://www.nhlbi.nih.gov/health/respiratory-distress-syndrome

Case 3.8

Zellweger Syndrome

COMPETENCY

- **BC4.8:** Interpret laboratory results of analytes associated with metabolism of Lipids

Case Scenario

A male infant was born at term. Labor and delivery were uncomplicated. After birth, he was noted to be floppy and had Apgar scores of 5. He required oxygen supplementation and was transferred to the neonatal intensive care unit. In the unit, he was persistently hypotonic with periods of apnea. He was noted to have a large anterior fontanelle, large forehead, and broad nasal bridge. He had transverse palmar creases and bilateral club feet. Liver was palpable 2 cm below the costal margin.

Laboratory studies revealed hyperbilirubinemia with a mild elevation in liver transaminases, serum very long chain fatty acid were found elevated.

QUESTIONS

Q.1. What is most probable diagnosis? What is biochemical defect in this clinical condition?

Q.2. What is the basis of your diagnosis? How you confirm your diagnosis?

Q.3. Enlist differential diagnosis of this clinical condition.

Q.4. What is the management in this patient?

ANSWERS

A.1. Child is suffering from Zellweger syndrome. It is an autosomal recessive disorder and also known as peroxisome biogenesis disorders (PBDs), which is a group of disorders characterized by the failure of the body to produce peroxisomes that function properly. ZSD develop due to changes (mutations) of one of 13 different genes (PEX gene) involved in the creation and proper function of peroxisomes (peroxisome biogenesis). Clinical signs and symptoms are summarized in **Figure 3.8.1.**

A.2. Typical clinical feature and detection of elevated very long chain fatty acids in blood are primary step to make diagnosis of ZSD. Genetic testing is available for ZSD. Next generation sequencing methods (sequencing millions of small fragments of DNA at the same time) are being used more frequently as a confirmatory test.

- Typical, distinctive and dysmorphic facies
- Hypotonia, visual and hearing impairment, development delay, seizure
- Progressive degeneration of brain/liver/kidney

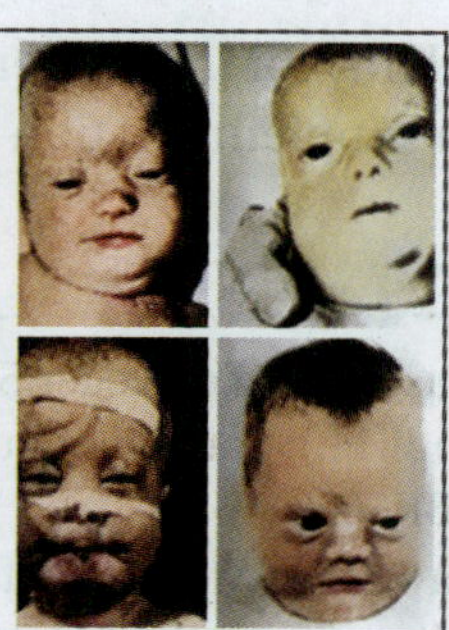

Fig. 3.8.1: Clinical presentation of Zellweger syndrome.

A.3. Symptoms of the following disorders can be similar to those of Zellweger spectrum disorders:

- Rhizomelic chondrodysplasia punctata (RCDP)
- X-linked adrenoleukodystrophy (ALD)
- Refsum disease

A.4. Zellweger syndrome is a rapidly progressive disorder with a high mortality rate. With no curative treatment available, treatment options are limited to supportive care to improve quality of life.

Various treatment modalities that have been tried include:

- *Docosahexaenoic acid:* This is a long-chain unsaturated fatty acid essential for myelination, brain, and eye development. The levels of docosahexaenoic acid are low in the plasma of patients with ZS. However, its replacement was not associated with improvement in neurological symptoms or visual disturbances in randomized controlled trials.
- *Lorenzo's oil:* Lorenzo's oil is a mixture of glyceryl trioleate and glyceryl trierucate, and its use was initially attempted in patients with X-linked adrenoleukodystrophy. It was shown to reduce VLCFA levels in plasma but did not affect disease progression in ZS patients.
- *Cholic acid:* This is 24 carbon bile acid, which is helpful in the absorption of fat-soluble vitamins. Due to liver dysfunction and lipoprotein synthesis impairment in patients with ZS, there is a deficiency of fat-soluble vitamins, and the use of cholic acid has been tried in other disorders of hepatic function. It has been approved by the US FDA for use in patients with ZS. However, there is little evidence regarding its efficacy.

Supportive measures include:

- Hearing aids or cochlear implants for hearing loss
- Ophthalmologist referral, cataract removal, and glasses for vision impairment
- Standard antiepileptic drugs for seizures
- Vitamin K supplementation for coagulopathy
- Cortisone for adrenal insufficiency

- Gastrostomy for insufficient calorie intake
- Vitamin supplementation for low levels of fat-soluble vitamins (A, D, E)

BIBLIOGRAPHY

1. Elumalai V, Pasrija D. Zellweger Syndrome. [Updated 2022 Aug 1]. In: StatPearls [Internet]. Treasure Island (FL): StatPearls Publishing; 2022. Available from: https://www.ncbi.nlm.nih.gov/books/NBK560676.
2. Rafique M, Zia S, Rana MN, Mostafa OA. Zellweger syndrome—a lethal peroxisome biogenesis disorder. J Pediatr Endocrinol Metab. 2013;26(3-4):377-9.

GIVE REASONS WHY

Q.1. TCA cycle is important for fatty acid synthesis.

Ans. One of the intermediate of TCA cycle is citrate which comes out from mitochondria to cytoplasm through tricarboxylic transporters. In cytoplasm it is cleaved by enzyme ATP depended citrate lyase.

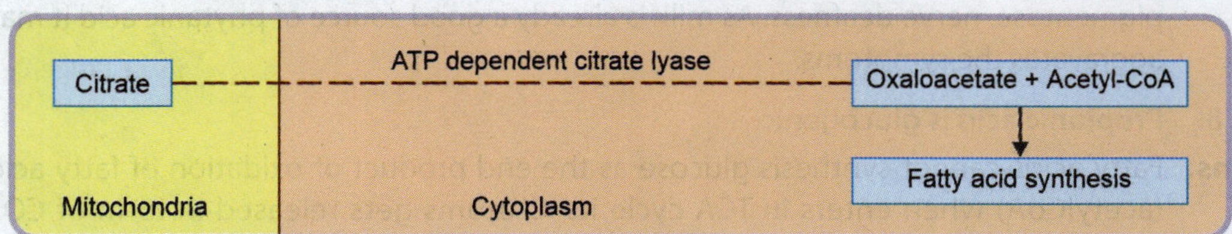

Q.2. PUFA is antiatherogenic but harmful if consumer in excess.

Ans. PUFA is a part of phospholipid (lecithin) is used for esterification of cholesterol during reverse cholesterol transport mechanism of HDL. This will help to bring the excess of cholesterol from extrahepatic tissues to liver for excretion through bile and that is how they have antiatherogenic property. A diet higher in omega-6 PUFA as compared to long-chain omega-3 PUFA may also promote insulin resistance, inflammation, and obesity.

Q.3. Defect in β-oxidation of fatty acids leads to hypoglycemia.

Ans. The end product of β-oxidation is acetyl-CoA which act an activator for pyruvate carboxylase (one of the key enzyme for gluconeogenesis), so if β-oxidation is defective there will not be synthesis of acetyl-CoA and decreased the rate of gluconeogenesis, result in hypoglycemia.

Q.4. Neurological manifestation in Zellweger syndrome.

Ans. Zellweger syndrome is characterized by defect in a gene which is responsible for formation of a protein "peroxin" which is needed for proper/correct assembly of peroxisomes, so defect in gene lead to defective organelle formation. In peroxisomes oxidation of very long chain fatty acids take place. This defect may lead to accumulation of VLCF (very long chain fatty acids) which further interfere with myelin sheath formation.

Q.5. Hyperemesis gravidarum leads to ketosis.

Ans. Hyperemesis gravidarum is excessive vomiting during pregnancy. This makes patient unable to eat anything and create a condition of starvation. Unavailability of glucose starts lipolysis in body and formation of excess at ketone bodies.

Q.6. Hepatosplenomegaly in Niemann's pick disease.

Ans. Niemann's pick disease is a lysosomal storage disease characterized by marked visceral accumulations of sphingomyelin due to absence or deficiency of sphingomyelinase there is accumulation of unesterified cholesterol in many tissues and storage of sphingolipids in liver, visceral organs and brain.

Q.7. Milk need to be avoided in Refsum disease.

Ans. Refsum disease is a metabolic error due to deficiency of α-hydroxylase (phytanic acid oxidase) so that there is no oxidation of phytanic acid. Phytanic acid accumulates in the tissues and results in various neurological symptoms like polyneuropathy, retinitis pigmentosa, nerve deafness. As milk is already a good source of phytanic acid it may aggravates the symptoms.

Q.8. Propionic acid is glucogenic.

Ans. Fatty acids cannot synthesis glucose as the end product of oxidation of fatty acid (acetylCoA) when enters in TCA cycle its 'C' atoms gets released in form of CO_2. However propionic acid (derived from oxidation of odd chain fatty acid) form succinyl-CoA and enters in TCA at a point after the CO_2 elimination and further in the form of oxaloacetate it can be channeled to gluconeogenesis.

$$CH_3CH_2-\overset{O}{\overset{\|}{C}}-SCoA \xrightarrow[\text{Propionyl-CoA carboxylase}]{HCO_3^- + ATP \;\; ADP + P_i \;\; \text{Biotin}} CH_3-\underset{COO^-}{CH}-\overset{O}{\overset{\|}{C}}-SCoA \xleftrightarrow{\text{Methylmalonyl-CoA epimerase}} CH_3-CH-COO^- \,(C{=}O,\ SCoA) \xleftrightarrow[\text{Methylmalonyl-CoA mutase}]{B_{12}} CH_2-CH_2-COO^- \,(C{=}O,\ SCoA)$$

Propionyl-CoA → D-methylmalonyl-CoA → L-methylmalonyl-CoA → Succinyl-CoA

Q.9. Dicarboxylic aciduria when β-oxidation is defective.

Ans. When β-oxidation is defective then rate of ω-oxidation increases. This takes place in microsomes, although it is a minor pathway but becomes dominant in defective β-oxidation. Terminal methyl (CH_3) group undergoes oxidation and produces dicarboxylic acid. So oxidation occurs at methyl end till the formation of dicarboxylic acids and these dicarboxylic acids are excreted in urine, known as dicarboxylic acid urea.

Q.10. B-complex vitamins are required for fatty acid synthesis.

Ans. Following B-complex vitamins are needed for fatty synthesis:

- Biotin as a co-enzyme for acetyl-CoA carboxylase.
- Pantothenic acid as integrate part of ACP (acyl carrier protein).
- Niacin: In the form of NADPH + H^+ which is required for reductive biosynthesis.

Section 4

Vitamins

- **Case 4.1:** Beri-Beri
- **Case 4.2:** Wernicke-Korsakoff Syndrome
- **Case 4.3:** Pellagra
- **Case 4.4:** Folic Acid Deficiency
- **Case 4.5:** Vitamin B_{12} Deficiency
- **Case 4.6:** Scurvy
- **Case 4.7:** Vitamin A Deficiency
- **Case 4.8:** Rickets
- **Case 4.9:** Vitamin K Deficiency

Give Reasons Why

Case 4.1

Beri-Beri

COMPETENCY

- **BC8.1:** Describe the Biochemical role of vitamins in the body and explain the manifestations of their deficiency

Integration with Pediatrics

- **PE12.7:** Describe the causes, clinical features, diagnosis and management of deficiency of B complex Vitamins

Integration with Medicine

- **GM24.3:** Discuss and describe the etiology, causes, clinical manifestations, complications, diagnosis and management of common vitamin deficiencies

Case Scenario

A 60-year-old female presented at our emergency department with 1-week febrile sense, progressive dyspnea, and generalized edema. A few days prior to this presentation, she had experienced several loose stools with intermittent abdominal pain localized to the right upper quadrant for 4 months.

She denied smoking or using illicit drug use, but confessed excessive and protracted alcohol consumption and a dietary pattern restricted to intake of only carbohydrates; specifically, eating only cookies without any intake of essential nutrients.

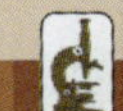

Laboratory Findings Reveal

- Aspartate transaminase (AST)—34 IU/L (8–20)
- Alanine transaminase (ALT)—34 IU/L (10–40)
- Total bilirubin 0.8 mg/dL—(0.2–1.2)
- Electrolyte levels, thyroid function test and cardiac enzymes like creatinine kinase (CK), CK-MB, and troponin-I were all within the normal range

QUESTIONS

Q.1. What is the most probable diagnosis in this case?

Q.2. Enlist the factors which can precipitate this deficiency disorder.

Q.3. Which investigation you require to confirm your diagnosis?

Q.4. What will be your treatment plan?

ANSWERS

A.1. Patient is most probably suffering from beri-beri. It is a severe and chronic form of thiamine (vitamin B_1) deficiency, characteristic clinical signs and symptoms are shown in **Figure 4.1.1**.

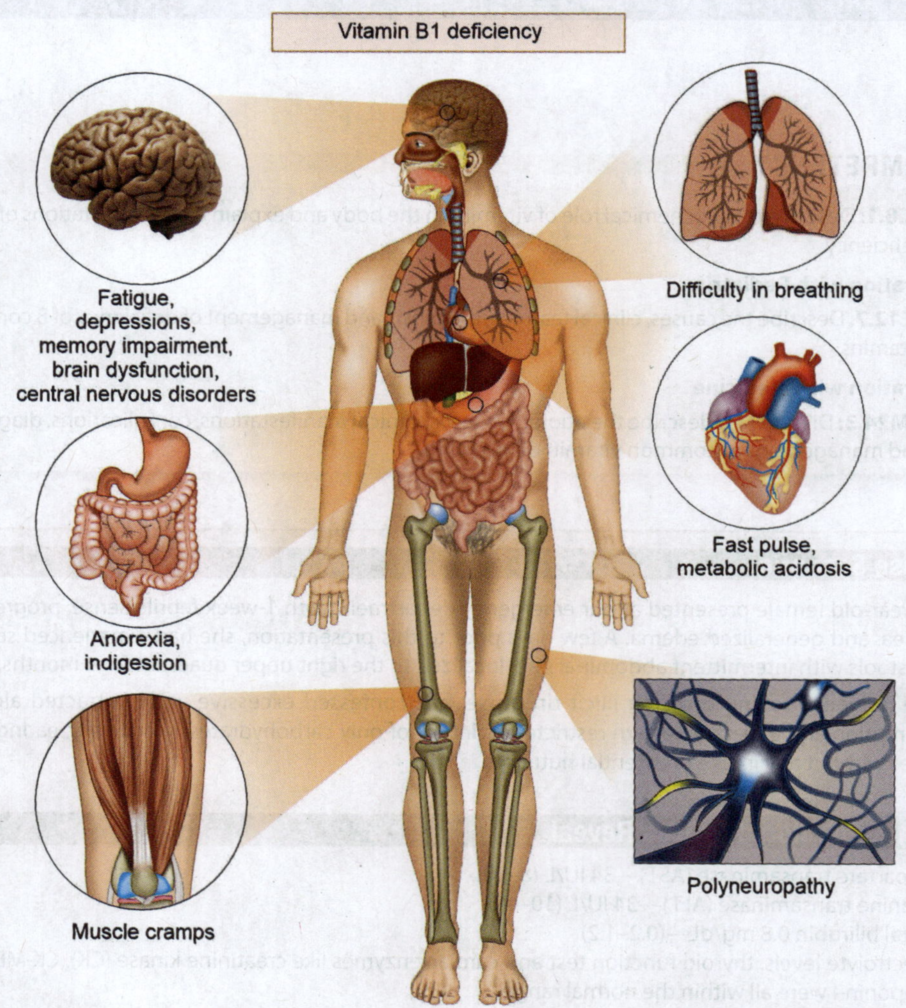

Fig. 4.1.1: Clinical presentation of vitamin B_1 deficiency.

The two main types in adults are:

Wet beri-beri: Wet beri-beri also known as shoshin beri-beri, cardiovascular beri-beri affects the cardiovascular system, clinical manifestation starts with vasodilation, tachycardia, a wide pulse pressure, sweating, warm skin, shortness of breath, and leg swelling and lactic acidosis. Later, heart failure develops.

Dry beri-beri: Dry beri-beri affects the nervous system, they affect predominantly the lower extremities, beginning with paresthesia's in the toes, burning in the feet (particularly severe at night), muscle cramps in the calves, pains in the legs. Continued deficiency worsens polyneuropathy and can result in muscle wasting.

Infantile beri-beri: Infantile beri-beri (thiamine deficiency) occurs mainly in infants breastfed by mothers with inadequate intake of thiamine, presents with sleeplessness, loss of appetite, vomiting, lactic acidosis, changes in heart rate, and enlargement of the heart.

A.2. Recommended daily allowance for thiamine is 1–1.5 mg/day and 0.5 mg/day additional per 1,000 kcal energy released from carbohydrate sources.

Precipitating Factors for Beri-Beri

Food habits: Diet consisting largely of highly refined carbohydrates as polished rice (oriental beri-beri), because thiamine is present in outer (aleurone) layers of cereals, diet-containing raw fish, raw shellfish, tea, coffee have thiaminase activity which destroy vitamin B_1.

Increased demand: Hyperthyroidism, pregnancy, lactation, strenuous exercise, or fever.

Decreased intake: Gastric or small intestinal resection, malabsorption syndromes hepatic insufficiency, diarrhea, hyperemesis gravidarum.

Interaction with other drugs: Alcohol, absorption is inhibited by thiamine analogues (such as metronidazole), diuretics (such as amiloride).

A.3. Laboratory investigations for confirmation of beri-beri are:

- Erythrocyte transketolase levels <0.75 (normal 0.75–1.30 IU/g Hb)
- Blood thiamine levels <2.5 (2.5–7.5 µg/dL)

A.4. Ensuring that dietary supplies of thiamine are adequate is important regardless of symptoms.

Start supplemental thiamine based on clinical manifestations.

- **For mild polyneuropathy:** 10 to 20 mg orally once a day for 2 weeks.
- **For moderate or advanced neuropathy:** 20 to 30 mg/day (as a single or divided dose), continued for several weeks after symptoms disappear.
- **For edema and congestion due to cardiovascular beri-beri:** 100 mg IV once-a-day for several days.

BIBLIOGRAPHY

1. Moonen M, Lancellotti P, Betz R, Lambermont B, Piérard L. Béribéri [Beri-beri]. Rev Med Liege. 2007;62(7-8):523-30.
2. Wiley KD, Gupta M. Vitamin B_1 thiamine deficiency. [Updated 2022 Jul 22]. In: StatPearls [Internet]. Treasure Island (FL): StatPearls Publishing; 2022. Available from: https://www.ncbi.nlm.nih.gov/books/NBK537204/

Case 4.2

Wernicke-Korsakoff Syndrome

COMPETENCY

- **BC8.1:** Describe the Biochemical role of vitamins in the body and explain the manifestations of their deficiency

Integration with Pediatrics

- **PE12.7:** Describe the causes, clinical features, diagnosis and management of deficiency of B complex Vitamins

Integration with Medicine

- **GM24.3:** Discuss and describe the etiology, causes, clinical manifestations, complications, diagnosis and management of common vitamin deficiencies

Case Scenario

A 60-year-old man presents with confusion, disorientation, and gait imbalance. Other than disorientation, bilateral paresis of gaze is noted. He has history of heavy alcohol intake for 15 years. He has progressive dementia. Physical examination shows weight loss and muscle wasting. There is no hepatomegaly.

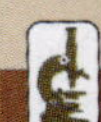

Laboratory Findings Reveal

- Blood glucose: 58 mg/dL (70–140 mg/dL)
- AST: 48 IU/L (8–20 IU/L)
- ALT: 38 IU/L (10–40 IU/L)
- CT head is negative for any tumor/injury

QUESTIONS

Q.1. What is the probable diagnosis? Explain the biochemical basis the cause of this condition.

Q.2. What is common cause for such a clinical presentation, how you can confirm your diagnosis?

Q.3. What is the plan of management of this patient?

ANSWERS

A.1. Patient is suffering from Wernicke-Korsakoff syndrome, precipitated due to deficiency of vitamin B_1. Clinical presentation of Wernicke-Korsakoff syndrome is summarized in **Figure 4.2.1**.

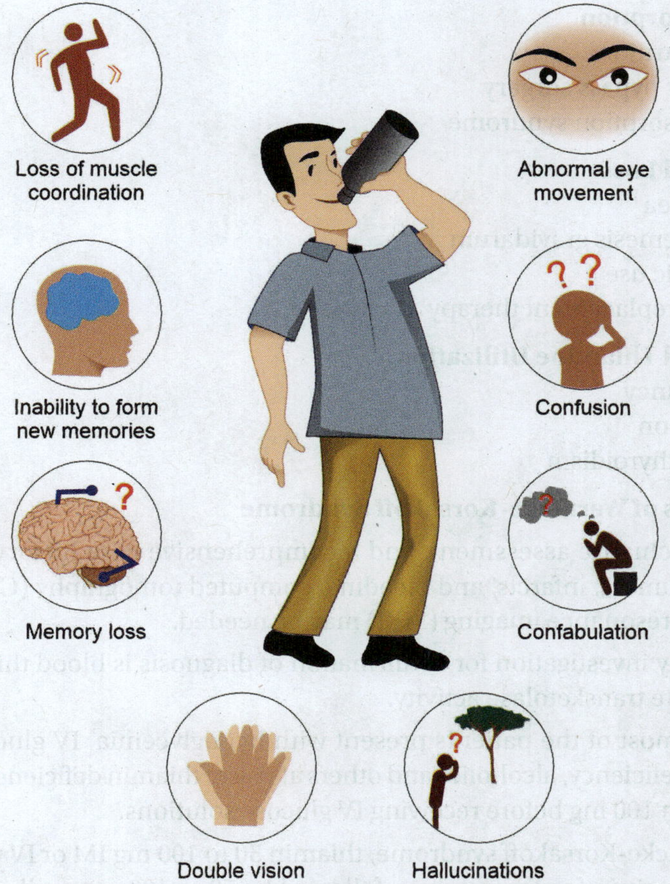

Fig. 4.2.1: Clinical presentation of Wernicke-Korsakoff syndrome.

Biochemical Basis of Clinical Signs and Symptoms

Mild thiamine deficiency presents with loss of appetite, fatigue, peripheral neuropathy, while is severe deficiency result in Wernicke encephalopathy—Korsakoff psychosis characterized by global confusion, ophthalmoplegia and ataxia (GOA).

Thiamin deficiency causes degeneration of peripheral nerves, thalamus, mammillary bodies, and cerebellum. Cerebral blood flow is markedly reduced, and vascular resistance is increased.

A.2. Chronic alcoholism with severe nutritional deficiency of thiamine is the most causes of such presentation, other common causes of thiamine deficiency.

Poor Intake

- Diets primarily high in polished rice/processed grains
- Chronic alcoholism
- Parenteral nutrition without adequate thiamine supplementation
- Gastric bypass surgery

Poor Absorption
- Malnutrition
- Gastric bypass surgery
- Malabsorption syndrome

Increased Loss
- Diarrhea
- Hyperemesis gravidarum
- Diuretic use
- Renal replacement therapy

Increased Thiamine Utilization
- Pregnancy
- Lactation
- Hyperthyroidism

Diagnosis of Wernicke-Korsakoff Syndrome

A full psychiatric assessment, and a comprehensive case history is essential. To rule out tumors, infarcts, and bleeding, computed tomography (CT) scanning and magnetic resonance imaging (MRI) may be needed.

Laboratory investigation for confirmation of diagnosis is blood thiamine level and erythrocyte transketolase activity.

A.3. Because most of the patients present with hypoglycemia, IV glucose can worsen thiamin deficiency, alcoholics and others at risk of thiamin deficiency should receive IV thiamin 100 mg before receiving IV glucose solutions.

For Wernicke-Korsakoff syndrome, thiamin 50 to 100 mg IM or IV twice a day must usually be given for several days, followed by 50 to 100 mg orally once a day until a therapeutic response is obtained. Anaphylactic reactions to IV thiamin are rare. Symptoms of ophthalmoplegia may resolve in a day; improvement in patients with Korsakoff psychosis may take 1 to 3 months. Recovery from neurologic deficit is often incomplete in Wernicke-Korsakoff syndrome.

BIBLIOGRAPHY

1. Akhouri S, Kuhn J, Newton EJ. Wernicke-Korsakoff syndrome. [Updated 2022]. In: StatPearls [Internet]. Treasure Island (FL): StatPearls Publishing; 2022. Available from: https://www.ncbi.nlm.nih.gov/books/NBK430729/
2. Covell T, Siddiqui W. Korsakoff syndrome. [Updated 2022 Jul 20]. In: StatPearls [Internet]. Treasure Island (FL): StatPearls Publishing; 2022 Jan-. Available from: https://www.ncbi.nlm.nih.gov/books/NBK539854/

Case 4.3

Pellagra

COMPETENCY

❖ **BC8.1:** Describe the Biochemical role of vitamins in the body and explain the manifestations of their deficiency

Integration with Pediatrics

❖ **PE12.7:** Describe the causes, clinical features, diagnosis and management of deficiency of B complex Vitamins

Integration with Medicine

❖ **GM24.3:** Discuss and describe the etiology, causes, clinical manifestations, complications, diagnosis and management of common vitamin deficiencies

Case Scenario

A 69-year-old woman with alcohol use disorder was brought to the emergency department with progressive disorientation, and disorganized speech. Two weeks before emergency episode patient had a history of watery diarrhea. On admission the patient was dehydrated, pale, lethargic, disoriented, she displayed symmetrical scaly rash with hyperpigmentation and hyperkeratinization in exposed areas of the skin.

QUESTIONS

Q.1. What is the most probable diagnosis, explain the biochemical basis of clinical signs and symptoms?

Q.2. How you confirm your diagnosis?

Q.3. What are the causative agents/precipitating factors of such clinical presentation?

Q.4. What is the line of management?

ANSWERS

A.1. Patient is most probably suffering from pellagra (vitamin B_3 deficiency disorders). Pellagra is an Italian word meaning rough skin. Major symptoms of pellagra are:

- **Dermatitis:** Early stages of deficiency is characterized by red erythema around ankles and face which on persistent deficiency may cause dark pigmentation around neck known as Casal's necklace.

- Diarrhea
- Dementia
- Death

Active form of niacin NAD+ and NADP+ are required as co-enzymes for more than 200 enzymes. Neurological symptoms in pellagra may be due to a serotonin deficiency caused by decreased tryptophan availability to the brain.

A.2. Confirmation of diagnosis of pellagra can be done by:

- Typical clinical sign and symptoms **(Fig. 4.3.1)**
- Dietary/medication history
- Blood level of vitamin B3 (niacin) found low
- Low levels of urinary excretion of N-methylnicotinamide and pyridone indicates niacin deficiency.

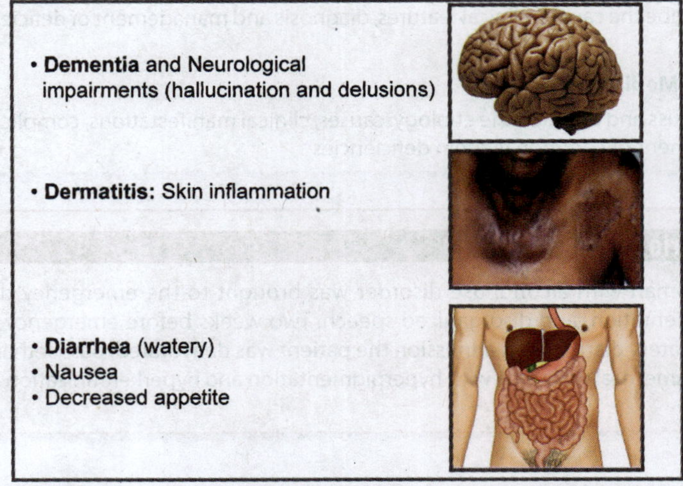

Fig. 4.3.1: Clinical presentation of pellagra (vitamin B_3) deficiency.

A.3. There are multiple causes of niacin deficiency:

- **Dietary deficiency of tryptophan:** Approximately 60 mg of tryptophan synthesizes 1 mg niacin.
- **Consumption of maize as staple diet:** In maize niacin is present in a bound form, which is unavailable for functioning.
- **Consumption of sorghum (jowar) as staple diet:** Sorghum is rich in leucine, which inhibits enzyme quinolinate phosphoribosyl transferase (QPRTase). This enzyme is required to convert niacin into active form NAD+.
- **Deficiency of pyridoxal phosphate (PLP) (vitamin B6):** This is the co-enzyme for kynureninase, one of the enzymes of tryptophan metabolism require for synthesis of niacin from tryptophan.
- **Antitubercular drug INH (isoniazid):** It inhibit formation of PLP.

- **Hartnup's disease:** This is a autosomal recessive disease characterized by defect in absorption of tryptophan from intestine.
- **Carcinoid syndrome:** Neuroendocrinal tumor of gastrointestinal tract, argentaffinoma—a tumor which secretes large amounts of the hormone serotonin from tryptophan. So, most of the tryptophan is used for serotonin synthesis leads to deficiency of niacin.

A.4. Management of Pellagra

Pellagra is treated by niacin. The WHO has recommended niacin to treat pellagra at 300 mg in divided doses for up to 4 weeks. Mucositis and diarrhea will improve within days, and neuropsychiatric changes improve in the first week. Skin changes may take a while to resolve totally.

For Prevention of Pellagra

Recommended dose for adults—10–15 mg/day.

(The WHO recommended intake is 6.6 niacin equivalents per 1,000 kcal for adults and children of 6 months or older).

BIBLIOGRAPHY

1. Pitche PT. Pellagre et érythèmes pellagroïdes [Pellagra]. Sante. 2005;15(3):205-8.
2. Prabhu D, Dawe RS, Mponda K. Pellagra a review exploring causes and mechanisms, including isoniazid-induced pellagra. Photodermatol Photoimmunol Photomed. 2021;37(2):99-104.

Case 4.4

Folic Acid Deficiency

COMPETENCY

- **BC8.1:** Describe the Biochemical role of vitamins in the body and explain the manifestations of their deficiency

Integration with Pediatrics

- **PE12.7:** Describe the causes, clinical features, diagnosis and management of deficiency of B complex Vitamins

Integration with Medicine

- **GM24.3:** Discuss and describe the etiology, causes, clinical manifestations, complications, diagnosis and management of common vitamin deficiencies

Case Scenario

A 26-year-old woman (gravida 4, para 3) was admitted at 31 weeks gestation with worsening fatigue and shortness of breath on exertion over a duration of 1 month. She reported about anorexia, pregnancy-related nausea, but denied any fever, night sweats or itching. There was no history of alcohol excess or any dietary restriction. All her previous pregnancies had been uneventful. On examination, she was pale and exhausted with no palpable lymphadenopathy or splenomegaly.

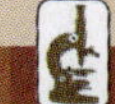

Laboratory Findings Reveal

Macrocytosis with a severe pancytopenia:

- Hemoglobin—7.2 g/dL (11.5–16.5 g/dL)
- MCV (mean cellular volume)—104 fL (80–100 fL)
- Platelets—15 × 10^9/L (150–400 × 10^9/L)
- Neutrophils—0.5 × 10^9/L (1.7–7.5 × 10^9/L)
- Vitamin B_{12} level—110 pg/mL (191–663 pg/mL)
- Serum folate—2.7 ng/mL (4.6–18.7 ng/mL)

QUESTIONS

Q.1. What is the probable diagnosis of patient? What may be the possible causes for this clinical presentation?

Q.2. Explain the biochemical basis of clinical signs and symptoms.

Q.3. How will you confirm the diagnosis?

Q.4. What will be the plan of management for this patient?

ANSWERS

A.1. Biochemical basis of clinical presentation in folic acid deficiency **(Fig. 4.4.1)**.

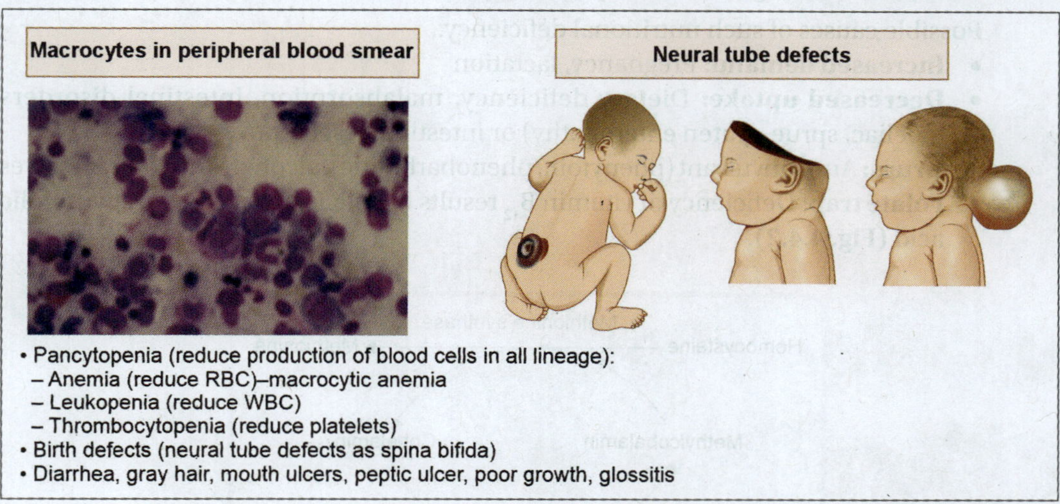

Fig. 4.4.1: Clinical presentation of folic acid deficiency.

Folic acid is essential in one carbon metabolism. As active form of folic acid, tetrahydrofolic acid acts as carrier of one carbon moieties for different metabolic reaction **(Table 4.1.1)**.

Table 4.1.1: One carbon moieties and their corresponding folic acid carrier.

Group	*Structure*	*Carried by*
Formyl	—CHO	N^5–formyl—THFA and N^{10}–formyl—THFA
Formimino	—CH=NH	N^5–formimino—THFA
Methenyl	=CH–	N^5, N^{10}–methenyl—THFA
Hydroxymethyl	$—CH_2OH$	N^{10}–hydroxymethyl—THFA
Methylene	$—CH_2–$	N^5, N^{10}–methylene—THFA
Methyl	$—CH_3$	N^5–methyl—THFA and methylcobalamin

One carbon metabolic reactions are essential in:
- Purine ring synthesis (C2 and C8 of purine ring)
- Pyrimidine synthesis (conversion of deoxyuridine monophosphate to deoxythymidine phosphate dUMP to dTMP)
- Transmethylation reaction
- Synthesis of choline, creatine, epinephrine

Deficiency of folic acid result in derange one carbon metabolism leads to:
- **Reduced DNA synthesis:** It affects rapidly diving cells like bone marrow (causes pancytopenia) intestinal mucosa (GIT upset) hair (hair loss). In pregnancy reduced DNA synthesis result in birth defects especially neural tube defects.

- **Hyperhomocysteinemia:** Accumulation of homocysteine result in increased risk of cardiovascular accidents.

A.2. Most probable diagnosis of this patient is folic acid deficiency.

Possible causes of such nutritional deficiency:

- **Increased demand:** Pregnancy, lactation
- **Decreased uptake:** Dietary deficiency, malabsorption, intestinal disorders (coeliac, sprue, gluten enteropathy) or intestinal resection
- **Drugs:** Anticonvulsant (phenytoin, phenobarbitone), alcohol, oral contraceptives
- **Folate trap:** Deficiency of vitamin B_{12} results in deficiency of free tetrahydrofolic acid **(Fig. 4.4.2)**.

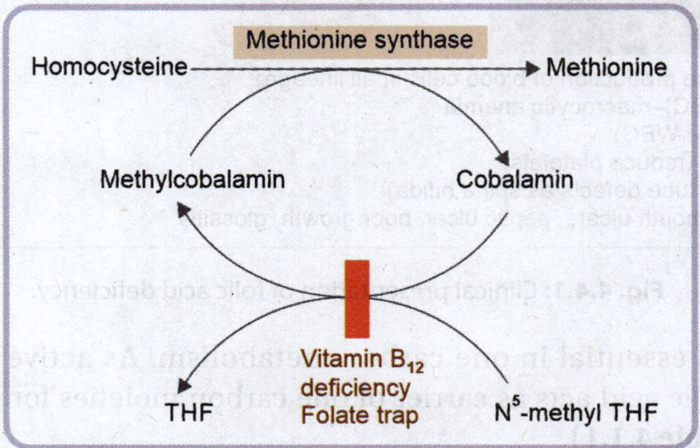

Fig. 4.4.2: Folate trap.

A.3. Confirmation of folic acid deficiency can be done by estimation of serum blood folic acid levels and histidine load test/FIGLU excretion test. During the metabolism of histidine FIGLU (formiminoglutamic acid) is synthesized as an intermediate which gives its formimino group to folic acid, but in case of folic acid deficiency, this process does not occur resulting in excretion of FIGLU in urine.

A.4. Therapeutic dose in 1 mg/day orally and always should be in combination with vitamin B_{12}.

Folic acid should never give alone in macrocytic anemia, as it will definitely decrease the symptoms of anemia but aggravate neurological symptoms of vitamin B_{12} deficiency.

BIBLIOGRAPHY

1. Donnelly JG. Folic acid. Crit Rev Clin Lab Sci. 2001;38(3):183-223.
2. Prabhu D, Dawe RS, Mponda K. Pellagra a review exploring causes and mechanisms, including isoniazid-induced pellagra. Photodermatol Photoimmunol Photomed. 2021;37(2):99-104.

Case 4.5

Vitamin B_{12} Deficiency

COMPETENCY

❖ **BC8.1:** Describe the Biochemical role of vitamins in the body and explain the manifestations of their deficiency

Integration with Medicine

❖ **GM24.3:** Discuss and describe the aetiology, causes, clinical manifestations, complications, diagnosis and management of common vitamin deficiencies

Integration with Pediatrics

❖ **PE12.7:** Describe the causes, clinical features, diagnosis and management of deficiency of B complex Vitamins

Case Scenario

A 59-year-old man with 6 months history of progressive loss of memory, disorientation, apathy, paranoid delusions, gait difficulties with falls, and urinary incontinence. He had suffered similar episode 3 years before, with a complete remission. Paleness and icterus in the sclera had been noted from last few weeks, the vegetarian patient had not consumed any food of animal origin for many years. Besides, his family only rarely ate fresh fruits or vegetables.

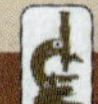

Laboratory Findings Reveal

Complete blood count shows pancytopenia, peripheral blood smear shows megaloblasts (large RBC) with hypersegmented neutrophils.

- Hemoglobin: 8 g/dL (12–16 g/dL)
- Vitamin B_{12}: 38 pg/mL (191–663 pg/mL)

QUESTIONS

Q.1. What is the probable diagnosis of patient? What may be the possible differential diagnosis for this clinical presentation?

Q.2. Explain the biochemical basis of clinical signs and symptoms.

Q.3. How will you confirm the diagnosis?

Q.4. What will be the plan of management for this patient?

ANSWERS

A.1. Patients is most probably suffering from vitamin B_{12} deficiency vitamin B_{12} (cobalamin) is a water-soluble vitamin that is derived from animal products such as red meat, dairy, and eggs. Intrinsic factor is a glycoprotein that is produced by parietal cells in the stomach and necessary for the absorption of B_{12} in the terminal ileum. Once absorbed, B_{12} is used as a cofactor for enzymes that are involved in the synthesis of DNA, myelin sheath and metabolism of odd chain fatty acids. As a result, B_{12} deficiency can lead to hematologic and neurologic symptoms. B_{12} is stored in excess in the liver. Clinical presentaion of vitamin B_{12} deficiency is summarized in **Figure 4.5.1**.

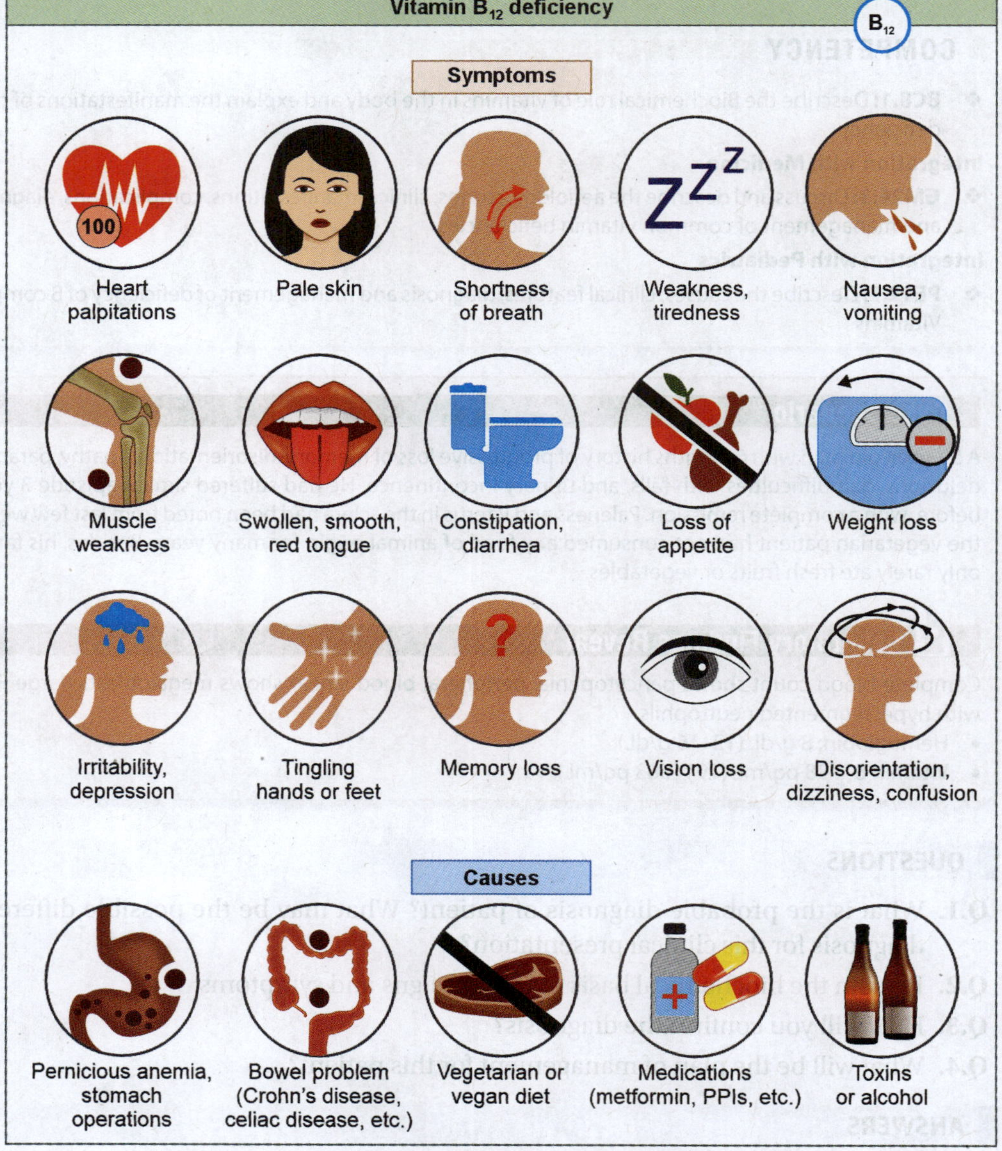

Fig. 4.5.1: Clinical presentation of vitamin B_{12} deficiency.

Vitamin B_{12} deficiency is primarily of three types:

1. **Autoimmune:** Autoimmune conditions like pernicious anemia where antibodies against intrinsic factor are produced. It will result in an inability of B_{12} to be absorbed by the terminal ileum.
2. **Malabsorption:** Patient with history of gastrointestinal surgery, gastric bypass surgery may be at risk for developing a B_{12} deficiency because parietal cells in the stomach produce intrinsic factor. In patients with normal intrinsic factor production, any damage to the terminal ileum, such as surgical resection due to Crohn's disease, will impair the absorption of B_{12} and lead to a deficiency. Other conditions like celiac disease or infection with the tapeworm *Diphyllobothrium latum*, may also result in a B_{12} deficiency.
3. **Dietary insufficiency:** Although vitamin B_{12} can be stored in the liver, but patients who have followed a strict vegan diet for long time may develop a B_{12} deficiency from a lack of dietary intake.

Differential diagnosis of vitamin B_{12} deficiency:

- Lead toxicity
- Syphilis
- HIV myelopathy
- Multiple sclerosis

A.2. Biochemical basis of clinical presentation is as follows:

- Decreased activity of methylmalonyl CoA mutase (isomerase) (vitamin B_{12} act as co-enzyme) leads to accumulation of methylmalonyl acid, as it cannot convert into succinyl-CoA resulting in metabolic acidosis, CNS depression.
- Decreased activity of methyltransferase (vitamin B_{12} act as co-enzyme) leads to:
  - **Demyelination:** Methylation of phosphatidylethanolamine and phosphatidylcholine is inadequate resulting in defective myelin sheath of nerves and neurological lesions.
  - **Homocystinuria:** Homocysteine cannot be converted into methionine leads to accumulation of homocysteine which predispose to increase cardiovascular events.
- **Folate trap:** Vitamin B_{12} deficiency results in trapping of folate in methyl THFA form resulting in deficiency disorders of folate co-exist.

A.3. Assessment of vitamin B_{12} deficiency can be assess by examination of peripheral blood smear and/or bone marrow morphology which shows megaloblastic anemia.

Other investigations are:

- Direct estimation of vitamin B_{12} levels in serum normal levels >145 pg/mL, depend on age and gender of person.
- Indirect methods are urinary levels of methylmalonyl acid and homocysteine levels, FIGLU excretion test.

A.4. Patients present with clinical presentation of macrocytic anemia should be treated with folic acid, vitamin B_{12} combination. Therapeutic dose of B_{12} is 500 to 1,000 micrograms by intramuscular injections.

BIBLIOGRAPHY

1. Ankar A, Kumar A. Vitamin B_{12} deficiency. [Updated 2022 Aug 12]. In: StatPearls [Internet]. Treasure Island (FL): StatPearls Publishing; 2022. Available from: https://www.ncbi.nlm.nih.gov/books/NBK441923/
2. Langan RC, Goodbred AJ. Vitamin B_{12} Deficiency: Recognition and Management. Am Fam Physician. 2017;96(6):384-9.

Case 4.6

Scurvy

COMPETENCY

- **BC8.1:** Describe the Biochemical role of vitamins in the body and explain the manifestations of their deficiency

Integration with Pediatrics

- **PE12.8:** Describe the RDA, dietary sources of Vitamin C and their role in Health and disease, clinical features of deficiency and management

Integration with Medicine

- **GM24.3:** Discuss and describe the etiology, causes, clinical manifestations, complications, diagnosis and management of common vitamin deficiencies

Case Scenario

A 13-year-old child who had been residing in a boarding school for the last 3 years was admitted to the hospital. On taking his history, he was found to have a poor appetite. His gums were swollen and tender. He was anemic and had complaints of fatigue, listlessness, muscular weakness and joint pain. Thorough examination of the patient revealed that he bruised easily and had edema and some subcutaneous hemorrhages on his limbs.

QUESTIONS

Q.1. What is the probable diagnosis and cause of disorder? Explain the biochemical basis of clinical symptoms.

Q.2. What is the line of treatment for this clinical condition?

Q.3. What is infantile Barlow disease?

Q.4. Explain biochemical basis of bony defects of scurvy. How they are different from vitamin D deficiency?

Q.5. List the antioxidant vitamins. Name the hematopoietic vitamins.

ANSWERS

A.1. Child is suffering from scurvy, which is severe vitamin C deficiency.

Vitamin C, or ascorbic acid, is an essential dietary nutrient. It plays a role in:

- Proper formation of collagen, the protein that helps give your body's connective tissues structure and stability

- Iron absorption
- Antioxidant action
- Wound healing
- Creation of neurotransmitters, like dopamine and epinephrine.

Deficiency of vitamin C leads to derangements of above-mention functions resulting in clinical signs and symptoms of scurvy shown in **Figure 4.6.1**.

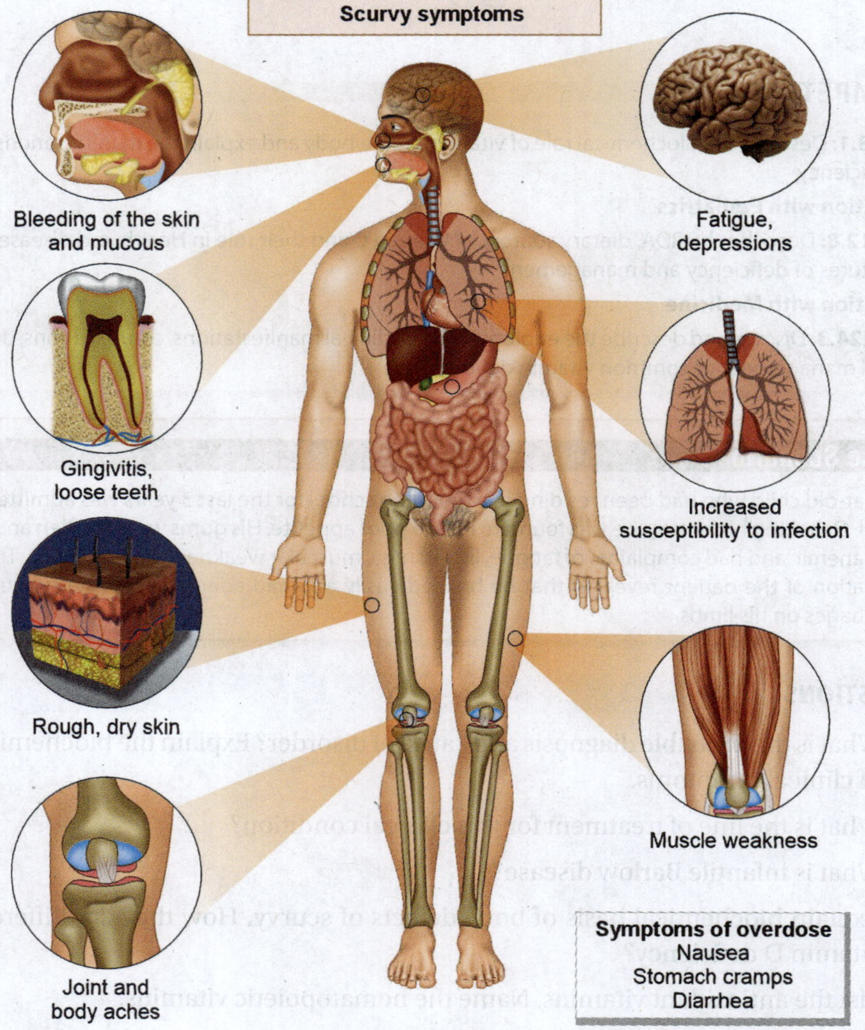

Fig. 4.6.1: Clinical presentation of scurvy.

A.2. Scurvy is fairly simple to treat. Direct replacement of vitamin C is standard, up to 300 mg for children and 500 mg to 1,000 mg for adults daily:

- Recommended daily dose of vitamin C to prevent deficiency disorders
- 75–90 mg of vitamin C per day (adult dose)

- Vitamin C is naturally found in many fruits and vegetables
- Rich sources of vitamin C (**Fig. 4.6.2**):
  - Guava
  - Gooseberry
  - Citrus fruits
  - Green leafy vegetables, broccoli
  - Berries, especially raspberries, strawberries, and blackberries pineapples and mango

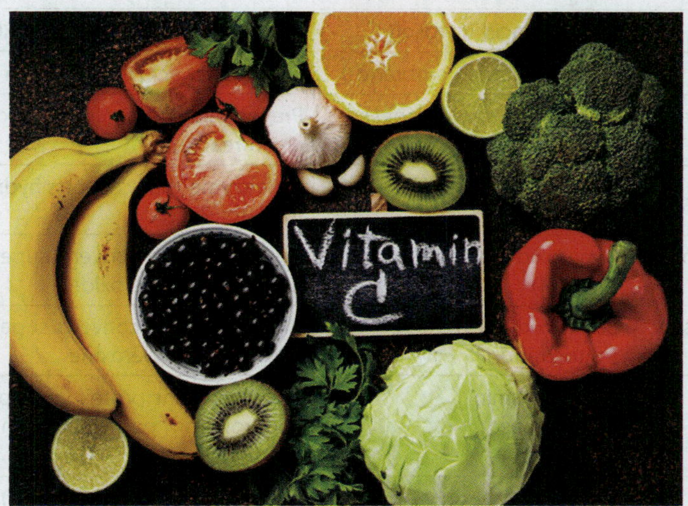

Fig. 4.6.2: Sources of vitamin C.

Air, heat, sunlight, cooking, canning and prolonged storage can greatly reduce the vitamin C content in foods.

A.3. Classical form of Barlow's disease or infantile scurvy, manifested by gingival lesions, hemorrhage, arthralgia, loss of appetite, and listlessness, broken bones and sores that will not heal.

Barlow disease also known as:

- Möller-Barlow disease
- Barlow's syndrome
- Cheadle-Möller-Barlow syndrome
- Moeller's disease
- Infantile scurvy

A.4. Formation of bone connective tissue (osteoid matrix) affected in vitamin C deficiency. In the connective tissues, major protein is collagen. Vitamin C is required for the post-translational modification of amino acids residues lysine and proline of collagen. This is required for H-bond formation between various amino acid residues, and cross-linking of polypeptides, which provide strength to the collagen while in vitamin D deficiency, there is mineralization of bone is defective.

A.5. Vitamins having antioxidants properties:
- Vitamin E
- Vitamin A
- Vitamin C
- Besides these vitamins, a few minerals are also having antioxidant properties shown in **Table 4.6.1**.

Table 4.6.1: Vitamins and minerals in antioxidant systems.

Nutrients	*Component (location in cell)*	*Functions*
Vitamin C	Ascorbic acid (cytosol)	Reacts with several types of ROS/RNS
Vitamin E	α-tocopherol (membranes)	Breaks fatty acid peroxidation chain reactions
β-carotene	β-carotene (membranes)	Prevents initiation of fatty acids peroxidation chain reaction
Selenium	Glutathione peroxidase (cytosol)	An enzyme that converts hydrogen peroxide to water
Copper and zinc	Superoxide dismutase (cytosol)	An enzyme that converts superoxide to oxygen and hydrogen peroxide
Manganese and zinc	Superoxide dismutase (mitochondria)	An enzyme that converts superoxide to oxygen and hydrogen peroxide
Copper	Ceruloplasmin (water phase)	An antioxidant protein, may prevent copper and iron from participating in oxidation reactions
Iron	Catalase (cytosol)	An enzyme (primarily in liver) that converts hydrogen peroxide to water

HEMATOPOIETIC VITAMINS

Vitamins those have hematopoietic properties:
- Vitamin B_{12}
- Folic acid
- Vitamin B_6 (pyridoxine)
- Vitamin C (ascorbic acid)

BIBLIOGRAPHY

1. https://ecosh.com/scurvy-vitamin-c-deficiency-symptoms-causes-risk-factors-and-treatment/
2. Léger D. Scurvy: Reemergence of nutritional deficiencies. Can Fam Physician. 2008;54(10): 1403-6.
3. Maxfield L, Crane JS. Vitamin C deficiency. [Updated 2022 Oct 12]. In: StatPearls [Internet]. Treasure Island (FL): StatPearls Publishing; 2022 Jan-. Available from: https://www.ncbi.nlm.nih.gov/books/NBK493187/

Case 4.7

Vitamin A Deficiency

COMPETENCY

- ❖ **BC8.1:** Describe the Biochemical role of vitamins in the body and explain the manifestations of their deficiency

Integration with Pediatrics

- ❖ **PE12.1:** Discuss the RDA, dietary sources of vitamin A and their role in health and disease
- ❖ **PE12.2:** Describe the causes, clinical features, diagnosis and management of deficiency/excess of vitamin A

Integration with Medicine

- ❖ **GM24.3:** Discuss and describe the etiology, causes, clinical manifestations, complications, diagnosis and management of common vitamin deficiencies

Case Scenario

A 25-year-old woman presented with a 4-week history of progressive loss of vision, first manifesting as night blindness. Additionally, the patient reported frequent severe episodes of diarrhea over the past month. Personal history reveals that she had three kids and youngest one of breastfed. Ophthalmological examination revealed severe bilateral corneal xerosis, bilateral Bitot's spots and inferior ulceration of the right cornea **(Fig. 4.7.1)**.

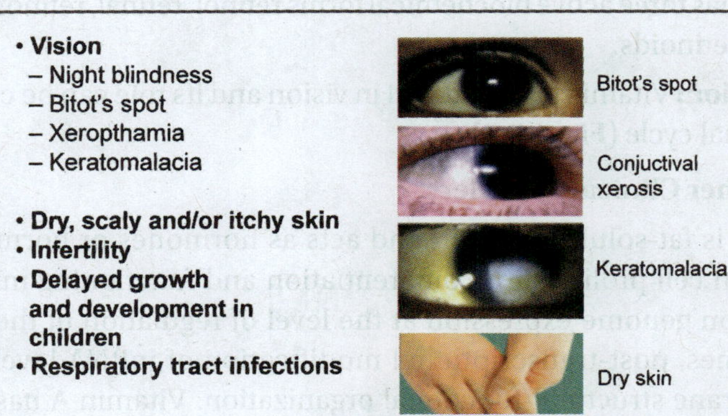

Fig. 4.7.1: Clinical presentation of vitamin A deficiency.

QUESTIONS

Q.1. What are the probable diagnosis and the causes of the such presentation?

Q.2. Explain biochemically the reason for clinical signs and symptoms.

Q.3. What are the appropriate first-line laboratory tests to narrow down the differential diagnoses?

Q.4. What dietary advice and treatment will you initiate for the lady? What measure should take to prevent such nutritional deficiency disorders?

ANSWERS

A.1. Patient is most probably suffering from vitamin A deficiency

Causes of Deficiency

- Increased demand: Pregnancy, lactation
- Decreased absorption: Diseases and conditions that impair intestine's ability to absorb fat can also cause vitamin A deficiency as:
  - Chronic diarrhea.
  - Celiac disease.
  - Cystic fibrosis.
  - Certain pancreatic disorders.
  - Bile duct blockage.
  - Zinc or iron deficiency.
  - Small bowel bypass or bariatric surgery.
  - Alcohol use disorder.
  - Intestine or pancreas surgery.
- Liver disorders

A.2. Biochemical basis of clinical signs and symptoms

Vitamin A has three active biochemical forms retinol, retinal, retinoic acid collectively known as retinoids.

Role in vision: Vitamin A is essential in vision and its role can be comprehended by Wald's visual cycle (**Fig. 4.7.2**).

Role in Other Clinical Disorders

Vitamin A is fat-soluble vitamin and acts as hormones or hormone's like factor. It effects on cell proliferation, differentiation and functioning might be due to its influence on genome expression at the level of regulation of the transcription of certain genes, post-transcriptional modification of mRNA levels, or changes in the membrane structural-functional organization. Vitamin A has antioxidant and anticancer properties. Clinical presentaion of vitamin A deficiency is summarized in **Figure 4.7.1**.

A.3. Diagnosis of vitamin A deficiency depend on complete ophthalmic examination and blood levels of vitamin A (normal level of vitamin A 25–50 μg/dL).

A.4. Treatment of Vitamin A deficiency

All case of vitamin deficiency should be treated urgently as vitamin A supplements (VSA) can reverse the condition if starts before involvement of cornea (keratomalacia).

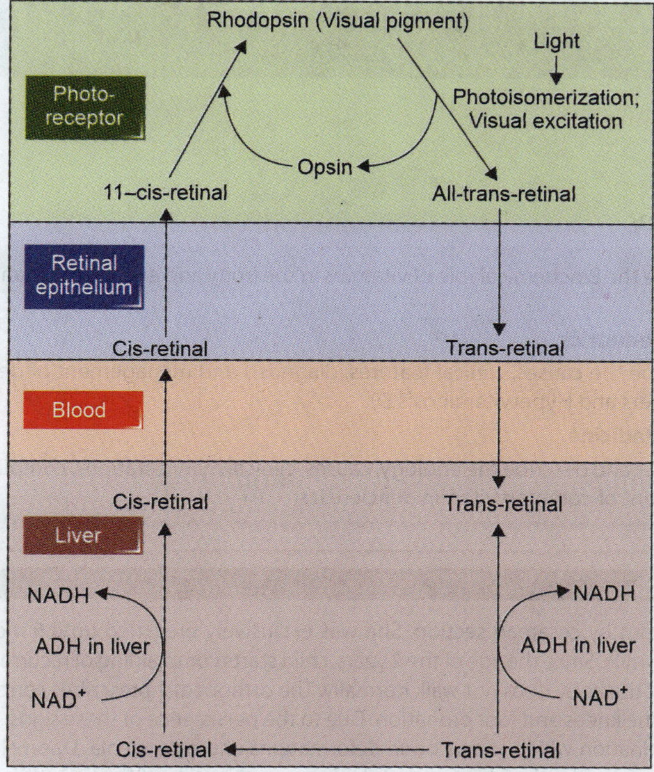

Fig. 4.7.2: Wald's visual cycle.

The WHO recommends treating xerophthalmia with VAS of 50,000 IU for children less than 6 months of age, 1,00,000 IU for children 6-12 months of age, and 2,00,000 IU for children more than 12 months of age daily for 2 days followed by an additional dose after 2 weeks.

Dietary Advice for Prevention

Vitamin A is exclusively found in animal diets, while beta-carotene (pro-vitamin A) found in vegetarian sources. The main food sources of beta-carotene are yellow, red and green (leafy) vegetables, such as spinach, carrots, sweet potatoes and red peppers, yellow fruit, such as mango, papaya and apricots.

BIBLIOGRAPHY

1. Hodge C, Taylor C. Vitamin A deficiency. [Updated 2022 May 15]. In: StatPearls [Internet]. Treasure Island (FL): StatPearls Publishing; 2022 Jan. Available from: https://www.ncbi.nlm.nih.gov/books/NBK567744/
2. Schoeff L. Vitamin A. Am J Med Technol. 1983;49(6):447-52.

Case 4.8

Rickets

COMPETENCY

- **BC8.1:** Describe the Biochemical role of vitamins in the body and explain the manifestations of their deficiency

Integration with Pediatrics

- **PE12.3:** Describe the causes, clinical features, diagnosis and management of deficiency/excess of Vitamin D (Rickets and Hypervitaminosis D)

Integration with Medicine

- **GM24.3:** Discuss and describe the etiology, causes, clinical manifestations, complications, diagnosis and management of common vitamin deficiencies

Case Scenario

A 5-year-old girl, born by cesarean section. She was exclusively breastfed until 6 months of age, then switched to formula milk. Since the age of the 2 years, child starts complaining of recurrent hip pain and the mother reports that the baby does not walk normally. The orthopedist prescribes corrective insoles as he noticed valgum of the knees and foot pronation. Due to the persistence of these signs, the girl undergoes a radiological examination which shows bone deformations and osteopenia. Upon clinical examination doctor notice a prominent forehead, valgum of the knees and brevity of the limbs **(Fig. 4.8.1)**.

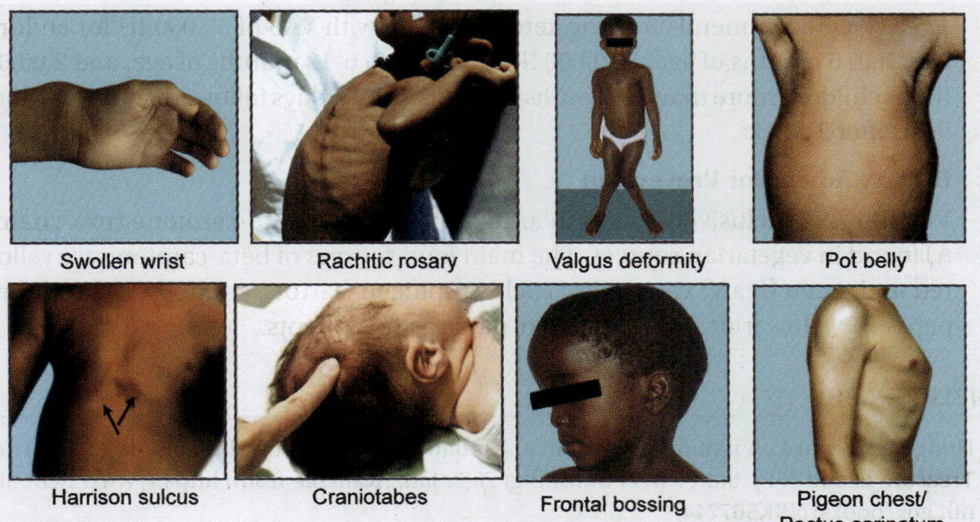

Fig. 4.8.1: Clinical presentation of rickets.

QUESTIONS

Q.1. What are the probable diagnosis and the cause of the disorder?

Q.2. Explain biochemically the reason for orthopedic deformities.

Q.3. What are the appropriate first-line laboratory tests to narrow down the differential diagnoses?

Q.4. What dietary advice and treatment will you initiate for the child?

ANSWERS

A.1. Patients is most probably suffering from rickets (vitamin D deficiency). Rickets is a nutritional deficiency disorder characterized by poor growth, insufficient mineralization, soft and weak bones which leads to bony deformities. In adults, similar conditions are known as osteomalacia. Clinical presentation of rickets is summarized in **Figure 4.8.1**.

Causes

- Dietary deficiency of vitamin D
- Nutritional deficiency of calcium or phosphorus
- Genetic causes, drug-induced rickets diphenylhydantoin and rifampicin
- Secondary to liver/renal diseases
- Celiac disease, inflammatory bowel disease, cystic fibrosis

Based on the biochemical profile, rickets can be classified into:

- Calcipenic—deficiency of calcium
- Phosphopenic rickets due to inhibited mineralization

A.2. Biochemical basis of clinical signs and symptoms

Vitamin D act as hormone which regulates various biochemical reaction in body (**Fig. 4.8.2**).

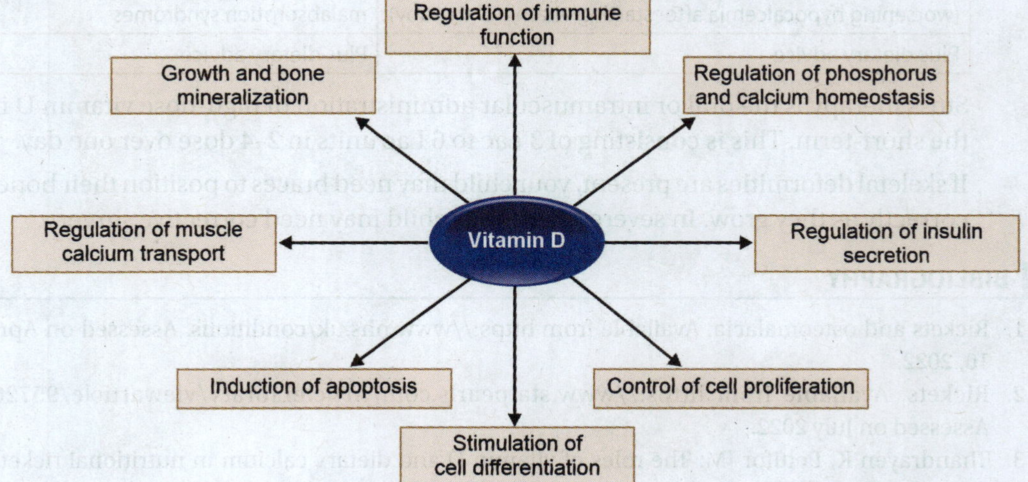

Fig. 4.8.2: Functions of vitamin D.

Most importantly vitamin D helps in regulation of calcium and phosphate in the body. These nutrients are needed to keep bones, teeth and muscles healthy.

Rickets is a childhood deficiency of vitamin D, which ultimately leads to defective mineralization, deranged calcium and phosphorus metabolism leads to characteristic bony deformities, bone pains, stunted growth, bone fractures, teeth deformities, and muscular weakness.

A.3. Diagnosis of rickets can be confirmed by laboratory investigations as:

- Blood calcium and phosphorus levels—below or normal levels
- Liver function test specifically serum alkaline phosphatase levels often increased
- Blood vitamin D levels—<15 ng/mL
- Radiological examination for bony deformities—widened, expanded growth plate
- Decrease in radio-opacity of cortical bone
- Deranged renal function tests.

A.4. Management of patients of rickets focuses on replacing the missing vitamin or mineral in the body advice for adequate sunlight exposure, dietary advice of food products high in vitamin D, such as fish, liver, milk, and eggs.

Calcium and vitamin D supplements can also be used to treat rickets **(Table 4.8.1)**.

Table 4.8.1: Treatment of nutritional rickets.

Vitamin D deficiency nutritional rickets	*Calcium deficiency nutritional rickets*
<1 m: 1,000 IU OD 3 months → 400 IU OD 1–12 m: 1,000-2,000 IU OD 3 months → 400 IU OD 1–12 y 2,000-6,000 IU OD 3 months → 600 IU OD Over 12 y: 6,000 IU OD 3 months → 600 IU OD	1,000 mg elemental calcium plus maintenance dose of vitamin D Maintenance doses of vitamin D:* <1 year: 400 IU OD
Stoss therapy for >3 m old can be tried if compliance is a concern	Over 1 year: 600 IU OD
Plus calcium supplementation 30–50 mg/kg/day of elemental calcium to avoid hungry bone syndrome (worsening hypocalcemia after starting vitamin D therapy)	*Higher doses for those at high risk for deficiency-antiepileptic medications, malabsorption syndromes
Plus dietary advice	Plus dietary advice

Stoss therapy is the oral or intramuscular administration of high-dose vitamin D in the short-term. This is consisting of 3 Lac to 6 Lac units in 2–4 dose over one day.

If skeletal deformities are present, your child may need braces to position their bones correctly as they grow. In severe cases, your child may need corrective surgery.

BIBLIOGRAPHY

1. Rickets and osteomalacia. Available from https://www.nhs.uk/conditions. Assessed on April 10, 2022.
2. Rickets. Available from https://www.statpearls.com/ArticleLibrary/viewarticle/95720. Assessed on July 2022.
3. Thandrayen K, Pettifor JM. The roles of vitamin D and dietary calcium in nutritional rickets. Bone Rep. 2018;8:81-89.

Case 4.9

Vitamin K Deficiency

COMPETENCY

- ❖ **BC8.1:** Describe the Biochemical role of vitamins in the body and explain the manifestations of their deficiency

Integration with Pediatrics

- ❖ **PE12.5** Describe the RDA, dietary sources of Vitamin K and their role in health and disease
- ❖ **PE12.6** Describe the causes, clinical features, diagnosis, management and prevention of deficiency of Vitamin K

Integration with Medicine

- ❖ **GM24.3:** Discuss and describe the etiology, causes, clinical manifestations, complications, diagnosis and management of common vitamin deficiencies

Case Scenario

A 2-months and 20-days male, presented with bleeding from the injection's sites of vaccines. His neonatal period was normal. He was exclusively breastfed. He had normal cardiorespiratory activity and normal vital signs.

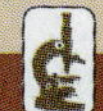

Laboratory Findings Reveal

- Hemoglobin: 7.4 g%
- Prothrombin time (PT): >100 s (11–13 second)
- Activated partial thromboplastin time (aPTT): 166 s (26–50 second)

QUESTIONS

Q.1. What are the probable diagnosis and the cause of the disorder? Add comment why such a deficiency disorder is common in infants.

Q.2. Explain biochemically the reason for clinical presentation.

Q.3. What are the appropriate first-line laboratory tests to narrow down the differential diagnoses?

Q.4. What dietary advice and treatment will you initiate for the child?

Q.5. What could be the other sites of bleeding?

ANSWERS

A.1. Child is most probably suffering from vitamin K deficiency. Fat-soluble vitamin K available in two form K1 (phylloquinone) comes from plants, especially leafy green vegetables like kale, collard greens, broccoli, spinach, cabbage, and lettuce and fruits like avocado, blueberries, grapes, apples. Vitamin K_2 (menaquinone) is naturally created in the intestinal tract by intestinal bacteria.

Causes of this nutritional deficiency:

- In adults fat malabsorption (celiac disease, cystic fibrosis, disorders of biliary tract, liver, gallbladder, and bile ducts), intestinal resection
- Prolong antibiotics
- Prolong anticoagulant therapy

Deficiency is more common in infants (**Fig. 4.9.1**), those who are on exclusive breast-feeding, whose mother on anticonvulsant therapy. Newborn infants are at increased risk for vitamin K deficiency for a variety of reasons:

- Breast milk is very low in vitamin K
- Vitamin K does not transfer well from a mother's placenta to her baby
- The liver of a newborn infant does not use the vitamin efficiently
- Newborns do not produce vitamin K_2 on their own in the first few days of life

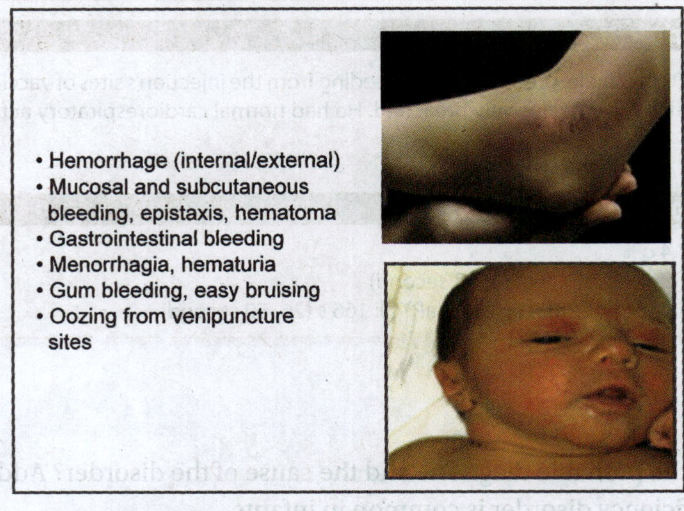

Fig. 4.9.1: Clinical presentation of vitamin K deficiency.

A.2. Biochemical basis of clinical presentation: Vitamin K plays an important role in blood coagulation. It is essential in activation of clotting factors 2, 7, 9, 10 through gamma carboxylation (post-translation modification of glutamic acid residues of these clotting factors).

A.3. Laboratory investigation for vitamin k deficiency is done by:

Coagulation screening tests: Prothrombin time (PT)—it is the most sensitive screening test to detect early or mild vitamin K deficiency. PT is prolonged and INR is elevated, but partial thromboplastin time (PTT), thrombin time, platelet count, bleeding time, and levels of fibrinogen, fibrin-split products, and D-dimer are normal.

Measurement of blood vitamin K levels (0.2 to 1.0 ng/mL) is confirmatory investigation.

A.4. Whenever, possible fat-soluble preparation of vitamin K (phytonadione) should be given intramuscularly. It can be given subcutaneously or orally and should be monitored with INR levels. The usual adult dose is 1 to 10 mg.

A.5. Other Sites

1. Intracranial bleeding
2. Gastrointestinal bleeding
3. Hemophilia

Water-soluble synthetic preparation is associated with vomiting, albuminuria, hemolytic anemia, hyperbilirubinemia. Injectable preparation should be avoided as it leads to flushing, breathlessness, anaphylactic reactions.

Prevention of Vitamin K Deficiency in Infants

0.5 to 1 mg IM (or 0.3 mg/kg for preterm infants) is recommended for all neonates within 6 hours of birth to reduce the incidence of intracranial hemorrhage due to birth trauma and of classic hemorrhagic disease of the newborn.

BIBLIOGRAPHY

1. Imbrescia K, Moszczynski Z. Vitamin K. [Updated 2022 Jul 11]. In: StatPearls [Internet]. Treasure Island (FL): StatPearls Publishing; 2022 Jan. Available from: https://www.ncbi.nlm.nih.gov/books/NBK551578/
2. Merrell BJ, McMurry JP. Folic acid. [Updated 2022 Apr 30]. In: StatPearls [Internet]. Treasure Island (FL): StatPearls Publishing; 2022 Jan. Available from: https://www.ncbi.nlm.nih.gov/books/NBK554487/

GIVE REASONS WHY

Q.1. Dark adaptation time increases in vitamin A deficiency.

Ans. In normal human being dark adaptation is due to duplex nature of our visual system. Two mechanisms are involved in vision.

Photopic vision: Above a certain luminance level (about 0.03 cd/m^2), the cone mechanism is involved in mediating vision.

Scotopic (night) vision: Below this level (about 0.03 cd/m^2), the rod mechanism comes into play.

Mesopic range: The range where two mechanisms are working together.

There is not an abrupt transition between the two mechanisms possible that is why whenever a person enters in a dark room from bright light (photopic to scotopic transition) it takes few minutes for proper vision.

In vitamin A deficiency scotopic vision is effected more because visual pigment rhodopsin is made up of retinal (form of vitamin A) and opsin protein. Vitamin A deficiency resulting in increased dark adaptation time followed by night blindness.

Q.2. Vitamin A is used to prevent acne.

Ans. Acne is the most common disease due to excess sebum formation and sebaceous growth. Vitamin A is known to reduce sebaceous secretions, so used in to prevent acne. It also prevents follicular hyperkeratosis.

Q.3. Markedly increase activity of alkaline phosphatase (ALP) in osteomalacia and bone disease.

Ans. Osteomalacia is softening of bone due to insufficient mineralization and patients are more prone to get fractures. Pre-β-ALP which contributes approximately 50% activity of total ALP is synthesized more and released from bone tissue. Bone specific alkaline phosphatase isoenzyme is elevated as a result of increased osteoblastic activity.

Q.4. Hypervitaminosis is seen with fat-soluble vitamins.

Ans. Fat-soluble vitamins are stored in liver and as they are not water-soluble, so, they cannot be excreted out in urine. So excess intake of fat-soluble vitamin causes toxicity or hypervitaminosis.

Q.5. Treatment of pregnant women with warfarin causes bone abnormalities.

Ans. Warfarin is a competitive inhibitor of vitamin K epoxide reductase. This enzyme is required for the carboxylation and consequent activation of vitamin K-dependent (VKD) proteins. Vitamin k is required for the gamma carboxylation of glutamic acid residues of osteocalcin. This protein is synthesized by osteoblast and required to bind the hydroxyapatite (CaPo4 H_2O) tightly to each other. Thus, vitamin K plays role in proper mineralization and that is why treatment with warfarin causes severe bone abnormalities.

Q.6. Hemorrhagic disease is commonly seen in premature infants.

Ans. Premature infants are more prone to develop vitamin k deficiency due to:

- Lack of intestinal flora to synthesize vitamin k
- Immature liver-leads to inadequate storage
- Low intake of vitamin k (exclusive breastfeeding)

Deficiency of vitamin k leads to deficiency of functional clotting factors as vitamin k is needed for γ-carboxylation of glutamic acid residues of clotting factors. It results in hemorrhagic disease, which may characterized as bruising tendency, ecchymotic patches, post-traumatic and nasal bleeding.

Q.7. Requirement of thiamine is increased with higher intake of carbohydrates.

Ans. Thiamine is needed for the activity of a group of enzymes related with carbohydrate metabolism.

- PDH—(pyruvate dehydrogenase complex)—it requires five coenzymes, thiamine (TPP), lipoic acid, pantothenic acid (CoA) riboflavin (FAD) and niacin (NAD+).
- α-ketoglutarate dehydrogenase—one of the enzyme of TCA cycle and activity is similar as PDH.
- Transketolase—enzyme of HMP shunt pathway.

Requirement of thiamine is increased 0.5 mg/1,000 kcal energy produced from carbohydrates.

Thiamine deficiency also results in lactic acidosis, it is because of decrease activity of PDH, causes accumulation of pyruvate which further reduces to form lactic acid.

Q.8. Polyneuritis is common in chronic alcoholics.

Ans. Alcohol abuse damages the lining of the gastrointestinal system and reduces absorption of nutrients. The toxic effects of alcohol can directly damage delicate nerve fibers and result in demyelination (damage to the protective sheath), results in disruption of electrical transmission in neuronal pathways, all of which can lead to neuropathy.

Q.9. Pellagra is seen among people where staple diet is maize and sorghum.

Ans. Pellagra occurs due to deficiency of niacin. In maize niacin is present but in a bound form. In sorghum leucine is present in excess amount, which inhibits enzyme quinolinate phosphoribosyl transferase (QPRTase) which is required to convert niacin into is active biochemical form.

Q.10. Pellagra is seen in Hartnup's disease.

Ans. Hartnup's disease is characterized by defective absorption and reabsorption of tryptophan from intestine and renal tubules respectively. This lead to deficiency of tryptophan. As in our body approximately 60 mg of tryptophan is required to synthesize 1 mg of niacin. So deficiency of tryptophan causes deficiency of niacin which ultimately leads to pellagra.

Q.11. Patient on anti-tubercular drug may develop pellagra.

Ans. Anti-tubercular drug INH leads to deficiency of pyridoxal phosphate (PLP). This co-enzyme is required for the activity of kynureninase, which is an enzyme of tryptophan metabolism, required to convert kynurenine into hydroxyanthranilic acid which finally convert into niacin. That is how anti-tubercular drug may lead to deficiency of niacin and causes pellagra.

Q.12. Unpolished grains have more nutritive value than polished one.

Ans. Unpolished grains are having a layer of aleurone which is rich in thiamine. Polishing of grains removes this layer causes thiamine deficiency.

Q.13. Vitamin B_6 (PLP) deficiency may cause convulsions.

Ans. PLP is a co-enzyme for decarboxylases. So, it is require to synthesize GABA (¥ amino butyric acid) from glutamate through decarboxylation. GABA is an inhibitory neurotransmitter, so deficiency of B6 (PLP) may causes convulsions.

Q.14. Consumption of raw egg causes deficiency of biotin.

Ans. In egg white, a protein avidin is present that has a great affinity for biotin (present in egg yellow). Avidin gets tightly bound with biotin and causes its deficiency. However, avidin is heat labile and boiling of egg can neutralize this inhibitory effect.

Q.15. Prolong use of antibiotics causes biotin deficiency.

Ans. Intestinal flora synthesizes biotin, excess use antibiotics destroys bacterial flora, lead to deficiency of biotin.

Q.16. Only two forms of vitamin B_{12} are functional in the body.

Ans. Four forms of B_{12} exist depending upon the type of molecules satisfied 6th valency of cobalt atom. This cobalt atom forms coordination complex with four porphyrin rings known as corrin ring, 5th valency with benzimidazole and 6th can be:

- Cyanide: Cyanocobalamin
- Hydroxy group: Hydroxocobalamin
- Adenosyl: Adenosyl cobalamin
- Methyl: Methylcarbylamine

First two forms are synthetic preparations, last two forms are found in human body.

Q.17. Folate trap is seen in cobalamin deficiency.

Ans. Active form of folic acid is tetrahydrofolic acid (THFA) which carries number of carbon moiety (during one carbon metabolism) which can be interchangeable except methyl THFA. Methyl group of THFA can only transfer its methyl group to the cobalamin B12 which finally transfer methyl group to homocysteine (Hcy) and convert it into methionine.

So if there is deficiency of vitamin B_{12}, folic acid remain trapped in methyl THFA. It is known as folate trap. To convert homocysteine into methionine **vitamin B_{12}** is needed. So deficiency of B_{12} causes hyperhomocysteinemia.

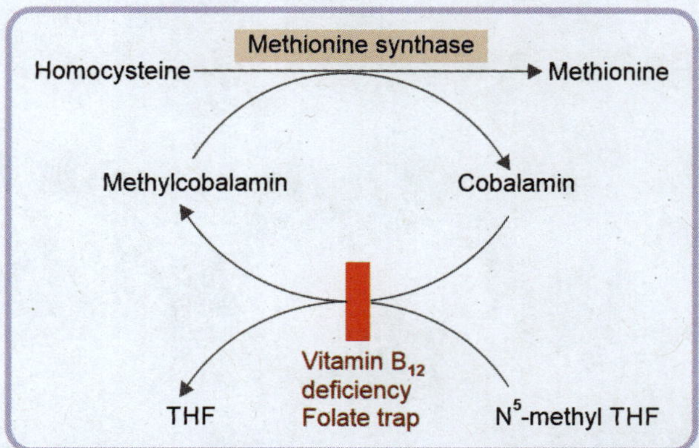

Q.18. Vitamin E reduces the selenium requirement.

Ans. Selenium act as an antioxidant mineral. It is the cofactor for glutathione peroxidase which is the key enzyme to reduce the oxidative stress of RBC.

Antioxidant action of selenium is complementary to vitamin E. So availability of vitamin E reduces the selenium requirement.

Q.19. Parathyroid hormone (PTH) level increase in chronic renal failure.

Ans. One step of activation of vitamin D takes place in epithelial cells of distal renal canalicular cells. So in case of CRF, this active form of vitamin D cannot be synthesized, which lead to hypocalcemia and decreased serum Ca^{+2} is a strong stimulator for PTH secretion.

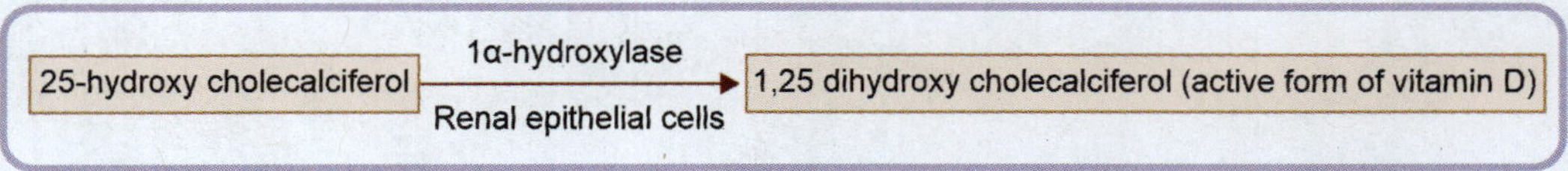

Q.20. Beri-beri is common in area in Japan.

Ans. In Japan, people consume raw seafood which contains an enzyme thiaminase, which cleaves the pyrimidine ring from thiazole ring of thiamine. So, dietary thiamine is not available and its deficiency leads to beri-beri.

Section

5 Minerals

- **Case 5.1:** Calcium Deficiency
- **Case 5.2:** Iron Deficiency
- **Case 5.3:** Copper Deficiency
- **Case 5.4:** Iodine Deficiency
- **Case 5.5:** Dental Fluorosis

Give Reasons Why

Case 5.1

Calcium Deficiency

COMPETENCY

- ❖ **BC9.1:** Describe the dietary sources, absorption, transport, and metabolism, Biochemical functions of Iron, Calcium and copper with its associated clinical disorders

Integration with Pediatrics

- ❖ **PE13.4:** Describe the RDA, dietary sources of Calcium and Magnesium and their role in health and disease, clinical features and management of deficiency states

Case Scenario

A 65-year-old man came to the emergency room of tertiary health care hospital with presenting complaint of abdominal pain and vomiting from last evening, associated with constipation over the previous week. Physical examination revealed the presence of persistent paresthesias and difficulty moving the arms, especially the hands. The patient's Trousseau sign was bilaterally positive.

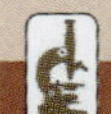

Laboratory Findings Reveal

- Serum calcium—4.9 mg/dL (9–11 mg/dL)
- Serum alkaline phosphatase—453 IU/L (40–130 IU/L)
- Creatine phosphokinase—5,267 IU/L (10–190 IU/L)
- Electrocardiogram at admission showed slightly prolonged QT interval (440 msec)

QUESTIONS

Q.1. What is the most probable diagnosis and common causes of such a clinical presentation?

Q.2. Explain biochemical basis of patient's clinical condition.

Q.3. Enumerate the laboratory investigations which can be helpful to confirm your diagnosis.

Q.4. What will be line of management for such clinical condition?

ANSWERS

A.1. Patient is most probably suffering from hypocalcemia. Clinical presentation of hypocalcemia is summarized in **Figure 5.1.1**.

- Muscle cramps, carpopedal spasm
- Paresthesia (tingling sensation) around mouth, fingers and toes
- Seizures
- Tetany
- Laryngospasm
- Cardiac rhythm disturbance (prolong QT interval)
- Chvostek's and Trousseau's sign

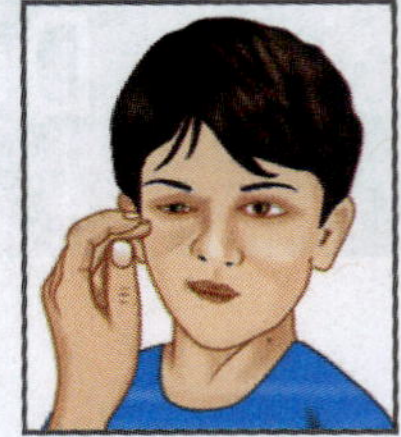
Chvostek's sign

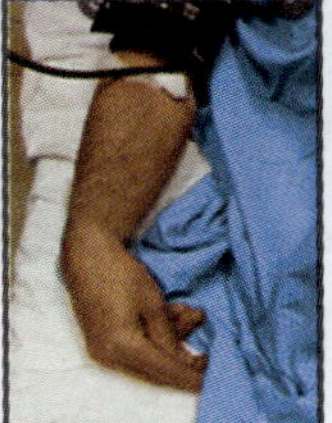
Trousseau's sign

Fig. 5.1.1: Clinical presentation of hypocalcemia.

Causes of hypocalcemia

- Inadequate vitamin D production and action
  - Nutritional deficiency
  - Lack of sunlight exposure
  - Malabsorption
  - End-stage liver disease and cirrhosis
  - Chronic kidney disease
- Inadequate PTH production/hypoparathyroidism
- Hyperphosphatemia
  - Phosphate retention in acute or chronic renal failure
  - Excess phosphate absorption caused by enemas, oral supplements
  - Massive phosphate release caused by tumor lysis or crush injury
- Drugs (intravenous bisphosphonate therapy or denosumab therapy/calcitonin/foscarnet)
- Rapid transfusion of large volumes of citrate-containing blood
- Acute pancreatitis.

A.2. Hypocalcemia can be acute and chronic in nature. Calcium causes excitation and contraction of muscles, upon getting the neural signal calcium is released from sarcoplasmic reticulum and activates ATPase, promotes the function of actin and myosin. Calcium is also required for nerve conduction. The hallmark of acute hypocalcemia is neuromuscular irritability, numbness and tingling in their fingertips, toes, perioral region.

- Tetany—may be manifested as neuromuscular irritability following signs may be present.
- Chvostek's sign—tapping over facial nerve causes facial contraction.
- Trousseau's sign—inflation of BP cuff for 3 minutes causes carpopedal spasm.
- Chronic hypocalcemia may have an entirely different presentation patient can present with seizure due to calcification of basal ganglia, dermal changes including dry skin, coarse hair, and brittle nails, atopic eczema, psoriasis. Changes in smooth muscle result in dysphagia, abdominal pain, biliary colic, wheezing, and dyspnea.

A.3. For the confirmation of diagnosis and management of hypocalcemia laboratory investigations which are helpful are as follows:

Basic investigations:

- Serum calcium (corrected for albumin): <8.7 mg/dL
- Magnesium: <1.5 mg/dL
- Electrolytes
- Creatinine
- Alkaline phosphatase: 40 IU/L
- Parathyroid hormone: <8 pg/mL
- 25-hydroxyvitamin D: <25 pg/mL
- Serum pH
- Complete blood count

Further investigations helpful in find cause of hypocalcemia:

- 24-hour urinary phosphate, calcium, magnesium, and creatinine
- Renal ultrasonography to assess for nephrolithiasis
- DNA sequencing to exclude genetic mutations
- Biochemistry in first-degree family members

A.4. Treatment of Hypocalcemia

Acute management of hypocalcemia: Intravenous calcium is given if serum calcium levels fall below 1.9 mmol/L, or ionized calcium levels are less than 1 mmol/L, or if patients are symptomatic. Intravenous calcium is given as one or two 10-mL ampoules of 10% calcium gluconate diluted in 50 to 100 mL 5% dextrose, infused over 5 to 10 minutes.

Precautions during intravenous calcium therapy:

- Intravenous calcium gluconate administered with a central venous catheter is preferable to avoid extravasation and irritation of the surrounding tissue.
- To avoid precipitation of calcium salts, phosphate and bicarbonate should not be infused with the calcium.
- Cardiac monitoring during intravenous calcium supplementation is necessary.
- Magnesium deficiency or alkalosis should be corrected if present.

Long-term management of chronic hypocalcemia: Oral calcium and vitamin D, and its metabolites are essential in management, addition to correction of hypomagnesemia.

BIBLIOGRAPHY

1. Fong J, Khan A. Hypocalcemia: updates in diagnosis and management for primary care. Can Fam Physician. 2012;58(2):158-62. Adapted from: Schafer AL, Shoback D. Hypocalcemia: definition, etiology, pathogenesis, diagnosis and management. In: Rosen CJ (Ed). Primer on the Metabolic Bone Diseases and Disorders of Mineral Metabolism, 8th edition. John Wiley and Sons., 2013. pp. 572-8.
2. Schafer AL, Shoback DM. Hypocalcemia: Diagnosis and Treatment. [Updated 2016 Jan 3]. In: Feingold KR, Anawalt B, Boyce A, et al. (Eds). Endotext [Internet]. South Dartmouth (MA): MDText.com, Inc.; 2000. Available from: https://www.ncbi.nlm.nih.gov/books/NBK279022.

Case 5.2

Iron Deficiency

COMPETENCY

- ❖ **BC9.1:** Describe the dietary sources, absorption, transport, and metabolism, Biochemical functions of Iron, Calcium and copper with its associated clinical disorders

Integration with Medicine

- ❖ **GM9.9:** Describe, develop a diagnostic plan to determine the etiology of anemia
- ❖ **GM9.16:** Communicate and counsel patients with methods to prevent nutritional Anemia

Case Scenario

A 32-year-old woman presents with chief complaint of increasing fatigue and dizziness for 2 weeks and mechanical fall at home. She was fully alert and oriented without any neurological deficits and was speaking in clear, full sentences. She had marked pallor with pale mucous membranes and conjunctiva. Peripheral blood smear shows erythrocytes with marked microcytosis, anisocytosis, and hypochromia.

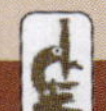

Laboratory Findings Reveal

- Hemoglobin—4.6 g/dL (12–16 g/dL)
- RBC count—2.8 M/mm^3 (4–5 M/mm^3)
- Serum iron—24 µg/dL (100–150 µg/dL)
- Serum ferritin—8 ng/mL (15–200 ng/mL)
- Total iron binding capacity (TIBC)—491 µg/dL (220–400 µg/dL)
- Vitamin B_{12}—860 pg/mL (191–667 pg/mL)
- Folic acid—12.8 ng/mL (4.6–18.7 ng/mL)

QUESTIONS

Q.1. What is the most probable diagnosis and causes of this clinical condition?

Q.2. What is the biochemical basis of signs and symptoms of patients?

Q.3. Enumerate the list of investigation which can be helpful to confirm your diagnosis.

Q.4. What will be that line of management in such clinical condition?

ANSWERS

A.1. Patient most probably suffering from iron deficiency anemia. Clinical presentation of iron deficiency anemia is summarized in **Figure 5.2.1**.

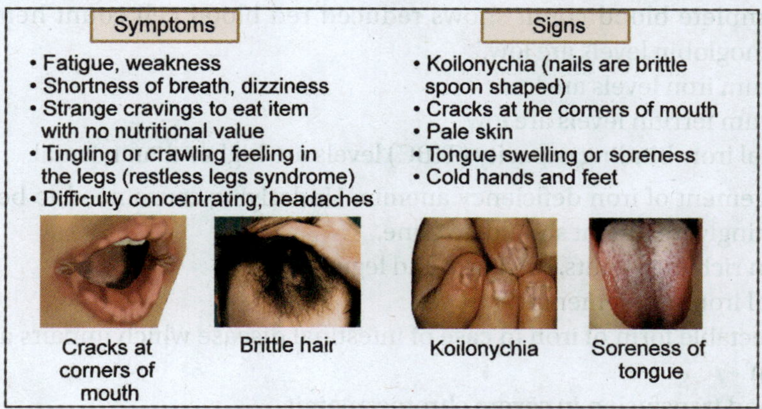

Fig. 5.2.1: Clinical presentation of iron deficiency anemia.

Common Causes of Iron Deficiency Anemia:

- Intestinal disorders (celiac sprue), gastrointestinal resection
- Zinc deficiency
- Vitamin C deficiency
- Increased demand (pregnancy, lactation)
- Chronic blood loss (gastrointestinal, menstrual, blood donation, hookworm, hemorrhoids)
- Intravascular hemolysis and hemoglobinuria.

A.2. Biochemical Basis of Sign and Symptoms of Iron Deficiency Anemia

Iron is essential for the production of hemoglobin, and hemoglobin is respiratory pigment responsible for oxygen transport to all tissues of the body. Iron deficiency will lead to decreased hemoglobin level and microcytic hypochromic anemia, which is the basis of most of symptoms. Beside that deficiency of iron will lead to decreased concentration of several iron-containing proteins such as myoglobin, cytochrome C, cytochrome oxidase, and xanthine oxidase.

Cytochrome and other sulfur containing proteins are integral part of electron transport chain and energy metabolism.

Iron acts as cofactor in synthesis of biogenic amines which acts as neurotransmitters. Iron is a cofactor for tyrosine hydroxylase and tryptophan hydroxylase, enzymes that are responsible for dopamine and serotonin synthesis. Altered metabolism of these neurotransmitter is the basis of change in behavior.

Iron is helpful in immune response against bacterial infection by activation of neutrophil and T cell.

A.3. In iron-deficiency anemia lab investigations which are helpful are:

- Peripheral blood smear shows microscopic, hypochromic red blood cells, reticulocytes are increased in number.

- Complete blood count shows reduced red blood cell count hematocrit and hemoglobin levels are low.
- Serum iron levels are low.
- Serum ferritin levels are low.
- Total iron-binding capacity (TIBC) levels are higher than normal.

A.4. Management of iron deficiency anemia: Underlying cause need to be known and accordingly treatment should be done.

- Iron rich diet—nuts, dry fruits and legumes
- Oral iron supplements
- Injectable form of iron in case of intestinal disease which impairs absorption of iron
- Blood transfusion in severe chronic anemia

BIBLIOGRAPHY

1. Chai AL, Huang OY, Rakocevic R, et al. Critical iron deficiency anemia with record low hemoglobin: a case report. J Med Case Reports. 2021;15:472.
2. Dallman PR. Biochemical basis for the manifestations of iron deficiency. Annu Rev Nutr. 1986;6:13-40.
3. DeLoughery TG. Iron deficiency anemia. Med Clin North Am. 2017;101(2):319-32.

Case 5.3

Copper Deficiency

COMPETENCY

❖ **BC9.1:** Describe the dietary sources, absorption, transport, and metabolism, Biochemical functions of Iron, Calcium and copper with its associated clinical disorders

Case Scenario

A 6.5-year-old boy was admitted with severe epistaxis and abdominal distension for 2 days. There was no history of bleeding from any other site, trauma or bowel disturbance. No past history of jaundice, hematemesis, abdominal distension or a bleeding disorder. His scholastic performance was satisfactory. One of his siblings had died at 6 months of age following severe epistaxis and mild jaundice with cause not known. Examination revealed low grade fever, severe icterus, pedal edema, a hepatomegaly and splenomegaly with ascites, ophthalmic examination revealed bilateral KF rings.

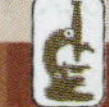

Laboratory Findings Reveal

- Hemoglobin—10.8 g/dL (12–16 g/dL)
- Total serum bilirubin—18.0 mg/dL (0.2–1.2 mg/dL)
- Serum SGOT—112 IU/L (8–20 IU/L)
- Serum SGPT—120 IU/L (10–40 IU/L)
- Serum alkaline phosphate—2000 IU/L (40–130 IU/L)
- PT—2 minute 9 sec (control 14 second)
- Serum ceruloplasmin level—04 mg/dL (14 to 40 mg/dL)
- Urinary copper level—100 mg/day (10 to 30 µg per 24 hours)

QUESTIONS

Q.1. What is the most probable diagnosis and cause of this clinical condition?

Q.2. What is the biochemical basis of such clinical condition?

Q.3. What is the line of management in this patient?

ANSWERS

A.1. Patient is suffering from Wilson's disease (hepatolenticular degeneration). Wilson's disease is an autosomal recessive disorder in which metabolic disorder of copper leads to its accumulation in the liver, brain, cornea and kidneys with consequent

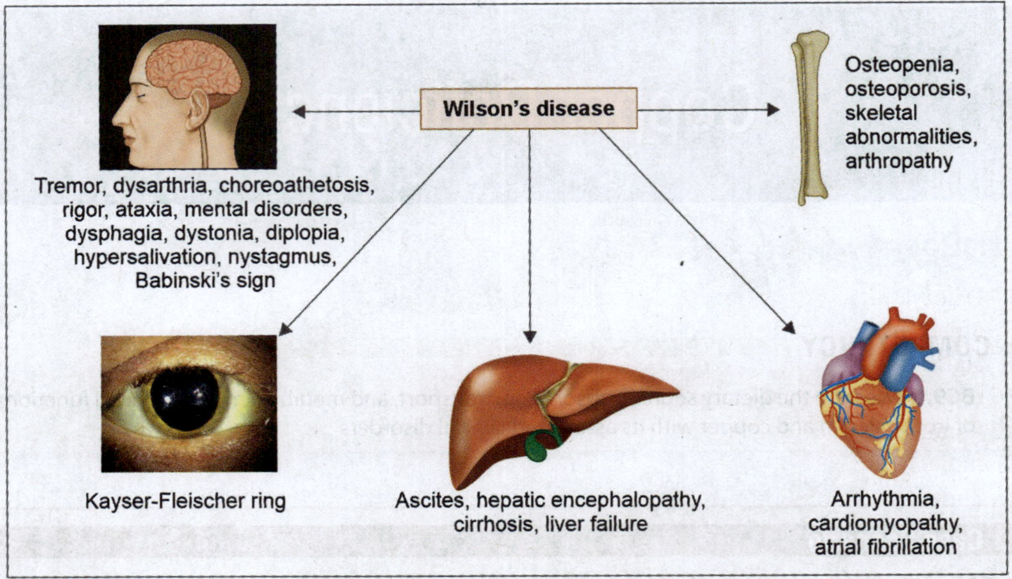

Fig. 5.3.1: Clinical presentation of Wilson's disease.

pathologic changes in those organs. Wilson's disease characterized by degenerative changes in the brain, cirrhosis and Kayser–Fleischer rings in the cornea **(Fig. 5.3.1)**.

Wilson disease was first described in 1912. Its incidence is 1 in 50,000–100,000. The gene concerned has been located on the chromosome region 13q14.

In children, the liver is primarily affected, so, it is referred as the hepatic form. As individuals age, neuropsychiatric symptoms become more significant called neurological form.

A.2. Biochemical basis of such clinical presentation: Possible hypothesis for accumulation of copper in this hereditary disorder:

- Disorder of ceruloplasmin metabolism caused by insufficient synthesis of normal ceruloplasmin, synthesis of functionally abnormal ceruloplasmin.
- Block of copper biliary excretion which is the consequence of the liver lysosomes functional defect.

Excess amount of copper release into circulation and accumulate in the brain, cornea, kidneys and bones, which causes adequate pathologic changes **(Table 5.3.1)**.

Toxic activity of copper is the consequence of its activity on enzymes, particularly on those with -SH group.

Table 5.3.1: Organs specific changes in Wilson disease.

Liver	Cirrhosis and hepatitis
Brain	Pathologic changes in the basal ganglia
Cornea	Kayser-Fleischer ring

A.3. The therapy of choice is penicillamine. If use it early, the result will be good and remission occurs in the majority of patients. It acts as general chelator and helps in urinary excretion of copper.

Trientine, zinc salts, tetrathiomolybdate, vitamin B_6, dimercaprol are other available treatment which are found beneficial.

BIBLIOGRAPHY

1. Dzieżyc-Jaworska K, Litwin T, Członkowska A. Clinical manifestations of Wilson disease in organs other than the liver and brain. Ann Transl Med. 2019;7(Suppl 2):S62.
2. Harharpreet Kaur, Kiranjit Kaur, Navneet Sharma, Kiran Kumar. Wilson's disease—a case report. International Journal of Contemporary Medical Research. 2019;6(7):G42-G44.
3. Kanitkar M, Joshi SN, Roy ND. Wilson's disease (A report of two cases). Med J Armed Forces India. 1994;50(1):63-65.
4. Zudenigo D, Relja M. Hepatolenticular degeneration. Neurologija. 1990;39(2):115-27.

Case 5.4

Iodine Deficiency

COMPETENCY

- **BC9.2:** Discuss Magnesium, Zinc and Phosphorus along with its clinical significance and discuss the functions of trace elements
- **BC14.19:** Explain the basis and rationale of Biochemical tests done and interpretation of laboratory results in Thyroid disorders

Integration with Pediatrics

- **PE13.3:** Describe the RDA, dietary sources of Iodine and their role in Health and disease, deficiency, and Goiter control program

Case Scenario

A 43-year-old hypertensive female migrated from north-eastern states of India, was referred by her primary care physician for evaluation for muscle weakness, weight gain, back pain, chronic constipation, cold intolerance and nodular swelling at thyroid. The patient had avoided consuming iodized salt ever since a diagnosis of hypertension. The patient had no family history of any thyroid disorder.

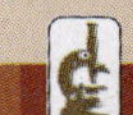

Laboratory Findings Reveal

- T3—0.1 pg/mL (2.3–4.2 pg/mL)
- T4—0.2 ng/dL (0.8–1.7 ng/dL)
- TSH—100 μIU/mL (0.34–4.25 μIU/mL)

QUESTIONS

Q.1. What is the most probable diagnosis and causes of this clinical condition?

Q.2. What is the biochemical basis of signs and symptoms of patient?

Q.3. Enumerate the list of investigations, which can be helpful to confirm your diagnosis.

Q.4. What will be that line of management in such clinical condition? What further complications can develop if patients remain untreated?

ANSWERS

A.1. Patient is suffering from iodine deficiency known as goiter. Patient is present with typical symptoms of hypothyroidism with swelling in neck region **(Fig. 5.4.1)**. Most common cause is nutritional deficiency of iodine in food or reduced intake of iodized salt.

- Swelling in neck
- Unexpected weight gain
- Fatigue and weakness
- Hair loss
- Dry and flaky skin
- Feeling colder
- Slower heart rate
- Learning and memory difficulties

Fig. 5.4.1: Clinical presentation of hypothyroidism.

Other causes of primary hypothyroidism

- Autoimmune thyroiditis (Hashimoto thyroiditis)
- Congenital hypothyroidism, absent or ectopic thyroid gland
- Silent thyroiditis (postpartum thyroiditis)
- Antithyroid drugs and cytokines
- Overexpression of deiodinase

Secondary hypothyroidism

- Hypopituitarism
- Hypothalamic disease
- Isolated TSH deficiency

A.2. Clinical signs and symptoms of hypothyroidism are summarized in **Figure 5.4.2.**

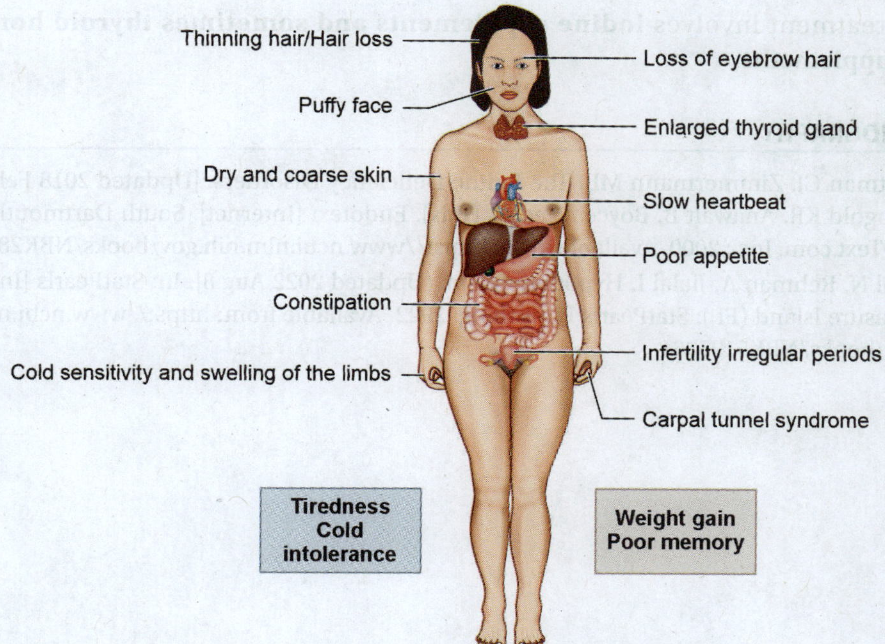

Fig. 5.4.2: Hypothyroidism.

Biochemical Basis of Signs and Symptoms

Reduced availability of dietary iodine result in decreased thyroid hormone production, as a result there is increase in TSH which stimulates thyroid follicular cells to synthesize more and more T3 and T4. It causes hypertrophy and enlargement of thyroid gland.

Puffiness of the face (myxedema) is a typical feature due to increased concentration of dermal glycosaminoglycans traps water, giving rise to skin thickening without pitting.

Weight gain is usually due to fluid retention.

Accumulation of fluid in other serous cavity results in pericardial effusion and in middle ear cavity causes conductive deafness.

Increase level of prolactin may cause alteration in libido and fertility.

Impairment of muscle functions results in Carpal tunnel syndrome is characterized by stiffness and cramps of muscles.

A.3. Laboratory diagnosis of iodine deficiency goiter (hypothyroidism) are as follows:
- Thyroid function test (T3, T4, TSH, Free T3, Free T4)
- Radiological assessment of swelling in neck
- Radioactive iodine uptake (RAIU)
- Thyroid scan—thyroid nodules and cystic lesions can be detected
- Autoimmune antibodies in autoimmune thyroiditis (Hashimoto thyroiditis)

A.4. Management of iodine deficiency hypothyroidism patients

Treatment involves **iodine supplements and sometimes thyroid hormone supplements.**

BIBLIOGRAPHY

1. Eastman CJ, Zimmermann MB. The Iodine Deficiency Disorders. [Updated 2018 Feb 6]. In: Feingold KR, Anawalt B, Boyce A, et al., (Eds). Endotext [Internet]. South Dartmouth (MA): MDText.com, Inc.; 2000. Available from: https://www.ncbi.nlm.nih.gov/books/NBK285556/
2. Patil N, Rehman A, Jialal I. Hypothyroidism. [Updated 2022 Aug 8]. In: StatPearls [Internet]. Treasure Island (FL): StatPearls Publishing; 2022. Available from: https://www.ncbi.nlm.nih.gov/books/NBK519536/

Case 5.5

Dental Fluorosis

COMPETENCY

- **BC9.2:** Discuss Magnesium, Zinc and Phosphorus along with its clinical significance and discuss the functions of trace elements

Case Scenario

A 12-year-old male patient was screened at the dental clinic for routine dental care. His wanted us to remove and/or minimize the noticeable brown/yellow staining of his teeth. The patient's desire to change the appearance of his teeth and improve his smile and thereby his confidence.

QUESTIONS

Q.1. What is the most probable diagnosis and common causes of such a clinical presentation?

Q.2. Explain biochemical basis of patient's clinical condition.

Q.3. What will be line of management for such clinical condition?

ANSWERS

A.1. Probable diagnosis is dental fluorosis. Dental fluorosis is due to ingestion of excess fluoride. In mild cases of fluorosis, there is presence of white opaque appearance of enamel along with increase surface porosity. Yellow to light brown staining is observed with moderate dental fluorosis. In case of heavy exposure few thick opaque bands as well patchy cloudy area appears on involved teeth **(Fig. 5.5.1)**.

High content of fluoride in drinking water and food supplements can cause fluorosis. Normal level of fluoride in drinking water is 0.5 to 1 ppm. When the level of fluoride is above 1.5 mg/L (1.5 ppm) in drinking water. It causes chronic intestinal upset, gastroenteritis, loss of appetite and loss of weight. Fluoride level more than 5 ppm results in mottling of enamel, stratification and discoloration. Level more than 20 ppm is toxic and causes osteoporosis and osteosclerosis.

A.2. Fluoride disturbs the normal morphology of enamel secretory cells, ameloblasts. After eruption, the enamel is exposed to mineral ions of the oral fluids, including fluoride, which can influence the composition of the outer layers of enamel. Matrix protein amelogenins remain retained in fluorosed enamel (fluoride reduces the proteolytic enzyme activity), this retention delays normal mineralization of enamel.

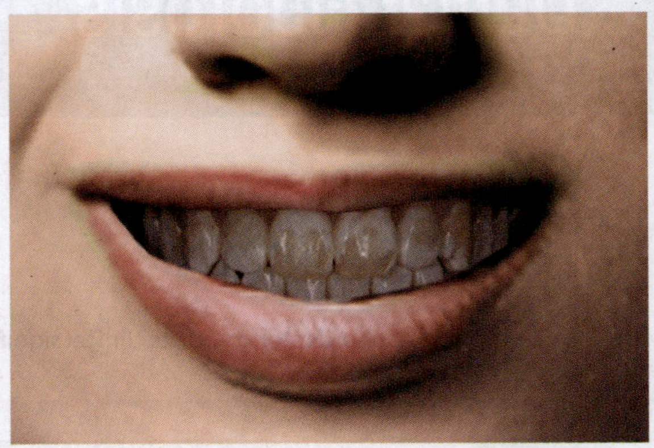

Fig. 5.5.1: Dental fluorosis.

A.3. Prevention and treatment

Dental fluorosis can be limited or prevented by following the 'recommended limits for fluoride exposure', suggested by US Environmental Protection Agency (USEPA).

Level of fluorosis is graded by a scale/index—TFI (Thylstrup and Fejerskov Index)

Based upon stages, treatment would be different:

- Mild (TFI = 1–3): Bleaching is recommended
- Moderate (TFI = 4–5): Microabrasion (outer affected layer is abraded from the tooth surface)
- Severe (TFI = 6–9): Aesthetic veneers or prosthetic crowns.

BIBLIOGRAPHY

1. DenBesten P, Li W. Chronic fluoride toxicity: dental fluorosis. Monogr Oral Sci. 2011;22:81-96.
2. Khandelwal V, Nayak UA, Nayak PA, Ninawe N. Aesthetic management of dental fluorosis. BMJ Case Rep. 2013.
3. Thylstrup A, Fejerskov O. Clinical appearance of dental fluorosis in permanent teeth in relation to histologic changes. Community Dent Oral Epidemiol. 1978;6(6):315-28.

GIVE REASONS WHY

Q.1. Why alkylating agents are prescribed for renal stone patients?

Ans. Composition of renal stones are mainly calcium oxalate, uric acid, calcium phosphate and calcium magnesium phosphate. Alkylating agents makes the urine alkaline and increases the solubility of renal stones, so that they can be excreted through urine.

Q.2. Sulfur is an important component of some vitamins.

Ans. Following water-soluble B-complex vitamins contain sulfur in their structure:

- Thiamine: Pyrimidine + thiazole (sulfur contain)
- Biotin: Imidazole + thiophene (sulfur contain)

Pantothenic acid: Sulfur is as such not an internal part of pantothenic acid, but along with beta-mercaptoethylamine (sulfur containing), it form an active form of vitamin that is CoA.

Q.3. Hyperparathyroidism causes demineralization of bones.

Ans. PTH increase number of osteoclasts, which secretes lactic acid in surrounding area causes solubilization of calcium. It also secretes collagenase which breaks the collagen protein of matrix and results in resorption of bone.

Q.4. Ferritin estimation is done in CKD (chronic kidney disease).

Ans. Inflammation associated with CKD increases ferritin levels independent of the body's iron composition, and thus ferritin estimation with other inflamatory markers is useful in CKD.

Q.5. Deficiency of copper causes anemia.

Ans. Copper is required for the following process:

- It is an integral part of key enzyme of heme synthesis that is ALA synthase.
- Ceruloplasmin is a copper containing protein which is required for the transport of iron by maintaining it into ferrous state. It facilitates normoblast (immature RBC) for uptake of iron.

Q.6. Fluorosis is more dangerous than caries.

Ans. Fluoride helps in prevention of dental caries. As in caries, acid formation (due to bacterial action on residual food in mouth cavity) causes removal of enamel and dentine to expose the root pulp. Topical applications of fluoride make a layer of fluorapatite on enamel and prevent its decay. But if the concentration of fluoride increases in the body it may result in various diseases.

Normal level of fluoride 40 µg/100 mL but in fluorosis the level increases >50 µg/100 mL, and it may results in—gastroenteritis, loss of appetite, mottling of enamel, discoloration of teeth, breakdown of bone matrix causing osteoporosis and osteosclerosis.

Q.7. Hemochromatosis is associated with diabetes.

Ans. There are two storage form of iron: (1) Ferritin and (2) Hemosiderin.

Hemosiderin is formed from proteolysis of ferritin and it is more water-insoluble. When [iron] is increased and it is beyond the capacity of ferritin to store, there is increased concentration of hemosiderin occurs known as hemosiderosis. This hemosiderin molecule starts accumulating in:

Hepatocytes—causes cirrhosis.

β-pancreatic cells—causes decreased release of insulin results in diabetes.

Subcutaneous tissue—yellow brown discoloration of skin known as hemochromatosis.

This combination of cirrhosis, diabetes and hemochromatosis is known as bronze diabetes.

Section

6 Enzymes

Case 6.1

Myocardial Infarction

COMPETENCY

- **BC2.4:** Describe and discuss the clinical utility of various serum enzymes in laboratory and their use as markers of various pathological conditions
- **BC2.5:** Interpret laboratory results of enzymes in various disorders
- **BC4.5:** Describe the metabolism of lipoproteins with brief overview of lipoprotein structure, their interrelations and relations with atherosclerosis
- **BC12.3:** Describe the role of oxidative stress in the pathogenesis of conditions such as cancer, complications of diabetes mellitus and atherosclerosis

Integration with Medicine

- **GM2.1:** Discuss and describe the epidemiology, antecedents and risk factors for atherosclerosis and ischemic heart disease
- **GM2.3:** Discuss and describe the lipid cycle and the role of dyslipidemia in the pathogenesis of atherosclerosis

Case Scenario

A 55-year-old man had a sense of tightness in middle of chest in early morning, accompanied by pain in the left arm. On examination the patient showed pallor, profuse sweating, his heart rate was increased (106/minute), blood pressure was low however it was a known case of hypertension from last 5 years. He went to hospital immediately, where ECG was done. Blood sample was taken for biochemical analysis. Patient revealed the history of chronic smoking, altered biochemical report of blood sugar and lipid profile.

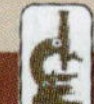

Laboratory Findings Reveal

- Creatine kinase—210 IU/L (10–190 IU/L)
- CK-MB—108 IU/L (5 to 25 IU/L)
- Cardiac troponin—72 ng/L (<30 ng/L)
- FBS—115 mg/dL (70–110 mg/dL)
- PP_2BS—180 mg/dL (<140 mg/dL)
- HbA1c—6.3% (<6%)
- Total cholesterol—226 mg/dL (up to 200 mg/dL)
- Triglycerides—180 mg/dL (<150 mg/dL)
- LDL—160 mg/dL (<100 mg/dL)
- HDL—30 mg/dL (>40 mg/dL)
- VLDL—36 mg/dL (<40 mg/dL)

QUESTIONS

Q.1. What would be the probable diagnosis? What are the causes and precipitating risk factors?

Q.2. What would be the pattern of onset, peak and disappearance of diagnostic markers in serum in this case?

Q.3. Explain the pathophysiology of the case.

Q.4. Define isoenzymes. What is the diagnostic significance of isoenzymes in such clinical condition?

Q.5. Enumerate the preventive measure for the development of such clinical condition.

Q.6. Name the enzymes which has therapeutic significance in this condition.

ANSWERS

A.1. Patients is most probably suffering from acute myocardial infarction (AMI).

AMI is an element of spectrum of clinical disorder known as acute coronary syndrome, classify as unstable angina, non-ST-elevation myocardial infarction (NSTEMI), ST-elevation MI (STEMI). Clinical presentation of myocardial infarction is summarized in **Figure 6.1.1**.

Potential precipitating factors of acute myocardial infarction:

1. Co-morbidities like hypertension and diabetes mellitus
2. Obesity and altered lipid profile
3 Acute emotional upset
4. Strenuous physical activity
5. Sudden changed position

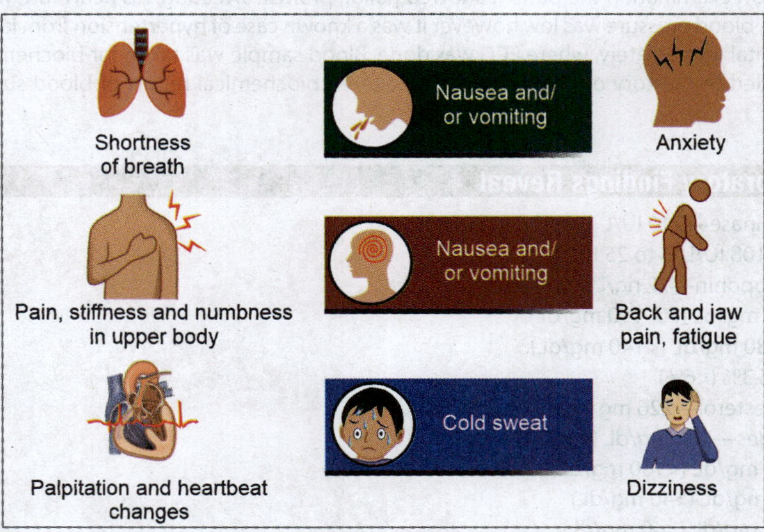

Fig. 6.1.1: Clinical presentation of myocardial infarction.

Risk Factors

- **Age:** Age > 65 years
- **Sex:** In men above 45 risk of heart attack increases greatly
- **Family history:** History of MI in parents or siblings
- **Lifestyle:** Lack of physical activity, diet high in sodium, sugar and fat tobacco, alcohol, drug abuse (cocaine amphetamines).

A.2. Pattern of onset, peak and disappearance of serum cardiac biomarkers as shown in **Figure 6.1.2**.

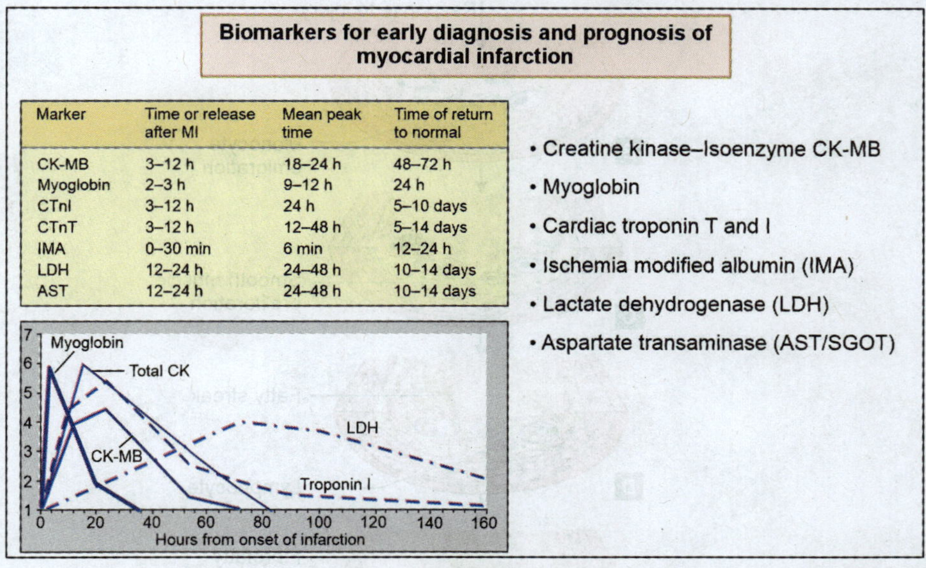

Biomarkers for early diagnosis and prognosis of myocardial infarction

Marker	Time or release after MI	Mean peak time	Time of return to normal
CK-MB	3–12 h	18–24 h	48–72 h
Myoglobin	2–3 h	9–12 h	24 h
CTnI	3–12 h	24 h	5–10 days
CTnT	3–12 h	12–48 h	5–14 days
IMA	0–30 min	6 min	12–24 h
LDH	12–24 h	24–48 h	10–14 days
AST	12–24 h	24–48 h	10–14 days

Fig. 6.1.2: Onset, detection and peak of cardiac biomarkers.

A.3. Myocardial infarction is a multifactorial disease. This is associated with sedentary life-style, diabetes mellitus and dyslipidemia (increase LDL and decrease HDL).

In the above case, patient is having hypertension and doing smoking on daily basis, and is having history of dyslipidemia and prediabetes which might act as an aggravating factors.

- Persistent hypertension and smoking caused damage to the endothelial lining.
- Hypercholesterolemia (LDL) particles get easily attach and enter into the intima through damaged endothelium.
- Hyperglycemia and oxidative stress causes glycation and oxidation of LDL.
- Such modified LDL triggers inflammatory response and signal for the lesion formation.
- Leukocytes migrate into the intima. Release of cytokines attracts macrophages and phagocytes.
- Phagocytes ingest lipid particles and become foam cells.

- Further smooth cells migrate from the media through internal elastic membrane to the intima and start accumulating there. This will result in formation of complicated atherosclerotic lesion which results in myocardial infarction **(Figs. 6.1.3A to E)**.

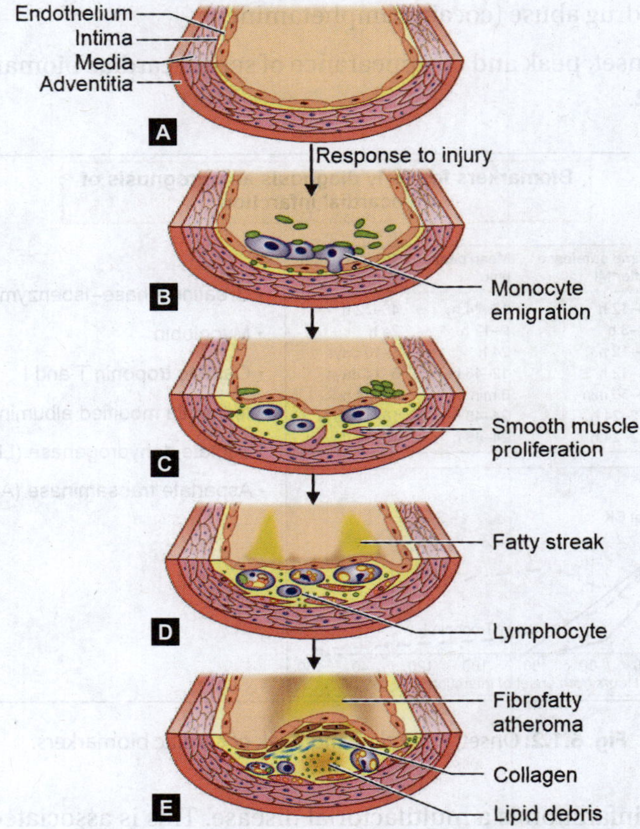

Figs. 6.1.3A to E: Atherosclerotic changes in myocardial infarction.

A.4. Isoenzyme: Multiple forms of same enzyme that catalyze the same chemical reaction, they can have different physical and chemical properties, electrophoretic motilities, amino acid composition and sequence.

Significance: Isoenzyme are more specific and valuable for diagnosis of particular clinical condition due to their location, tissue or organ specificity.

A.5. Management for myocardial infarction include lifestyle modification (avoid cigarette and excess sucrose, regular moderate exercise) other preventive measures which are useful as:

- Avoid trans-fatty acids intake
- Reduces dietary cholesterol
- Antioxidant vitamins should be included in diet

- PUFA (the optimal ratio for omega 6 to omega 3 = 4:1) should be included in diet.
- Medications such as statins, which are hypolipidemic drugs, act as competitive inhibitors of HMG-CoA reductase, the key enzyme involved in cholesterol synthesis.
  - Bile acid binding resins
  - Nicotinic acid which inhibit lipolysis, decreases VLDL
  - Fibric acid which increases β-oxidation of fatty acids

A.6. Streptokinase and urokinase are the enzymes of therapeutic significance as they are useful in lysis of fibrin clot in coronary artery.

BIBLIOGRAPHY

1. Lu L, Liu M, Sun R, Zheng Y, Zhang P. Myocardial infarction: Symptoms and treatments. Cell Biochem Biophys. 2015;72(3):865-7.
2. Smith M, Little WC. Potential precipitating factors of the onset of myocardial infarction. Am J Med Sci. 1992;303(3):141-4.

Case 6.2

Acute Hepatic Injury: Paracetamol Poisoning

COMPETENCY

❖ **BC2.3:** Describe and discuss enzyme Inhibition and role of enzymes or drugs as Inhibitors, and enzymes as therapeutic agents

Integration with Medicine

❖ **GM5.6:** Enumerate and describe the causes and pathophysiology of drug induced liver injury

Case Scenario

A 36-year-old male presented with severe abdominal pain and vomiting. On examination all vitals are stable, he seems to be disoriented. History reveals that patient consumes large dose of acetaminophen (paracetamol) off and on without doctor's prescription **(Fig. 6.2.1)**.

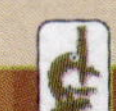

Laboratory Findings Reveal

- Serum SGOT—180 IU/L (8–20 IU/L)
- Serum SGPT—168 IU/L (10–40 IU/L)
- Alkaline phosphate—280 IU/L (40–130 IU/L)

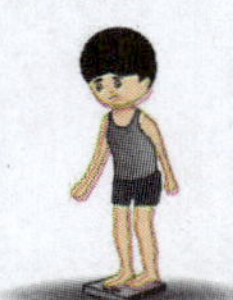

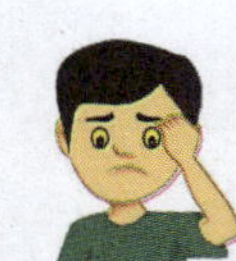

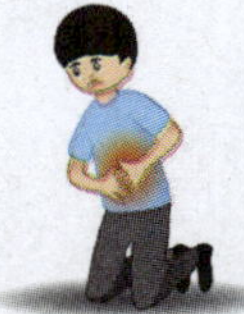

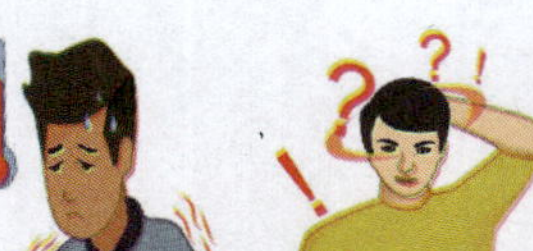

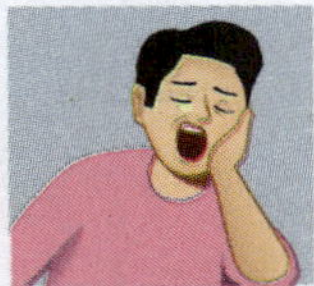

Fig. 6.2.1: Clinical presentation of acute liver injury.

QUESTIONS

Q.1. What is the most probable diagnosis of this patient? What are the other laboratory investigations which can be helpful to assess the severity of this clinical condition?

Q.2. Enumerate the list of other drugs, where overdose can lead to similar clinical presentation.

Q.3. Enlist few novel biomarkers which can be helpful in early diagnosis and prognosis of such drug overdose condition.

ANSWERS

A.1. Patients is suffering from drug-induced hepatotoxicity. Drug-induced liver injury (DILI) is of two types:

1. Direct (intrinsic toxicity)—dose dependent, typical example is liver injury by paracetamol
2. Indirect (idiosyncratic)—rare, unpredictable, occur at therapeutic doses, majority of drug induced liver injuries comes under this category.

Other important laboratory investigations are:

- Complete liver function tests
- Prothrombin time/INR
- Complete blood count

Complete blood count, low platelet count, anemia with high mean corpuscular volume (MCV), low lymphocyte with raised neutrophil count.

Elevated erythrocyte sedimentation rate.

Elevated prothrombin time (international normalized ratio, INR).

Elevated INR with low albumin suggests advanced liver disease.

A.2. There are more than 300 drugs which results in drug-induced liver injury (DILI). In India, anti-tuberculous drugs (58%), anti-epileptics (11%), olanzapine (5%), and dapsone (5%) are the most common causes.

While 10 most frequently implicated hepatotoxic drugs are amoxicillin-clavulanate, flucloxacillin, erythromycin, diclofenac, sulfamethoxazole/trimethoprim, isoniazid, disulfiram, ibuprofen and flutamide.

A.3. Few novel biomarker available for specific liver injuries are as follows:

- *MicroRNA-122:* The circulating microRNAs, miR-122 and miR-192 are hepato-specific. MicroRNA-122 is an early marker of hepatic damage (viral, alcohol, toxic). In paracetamol toxicity miR-122 is more sensitive and increased earlier than transaminases.
- *Cytokeratin 18:* It is released in hepatocyte necrosis, increase early in hepatic toxicity.
- *Glutamate dehydrogenase (GLDH):* Liver specific enzyme.

- Macrophage colony-stimulating factor receptor 1 (MSCFR1): It is a marker of immune system activation, specific for idiosyncratic drug reactions, not useful in evaluation of paracetamol liver injury.

BIBLIOGRAPHY

1. Lucy M, Dominique L. Drug-induced Liver Injury: Biomarkers, Requirements, Candidates, and Validation. Frontiers in Pharmacology. 2019;10.
2. Yoon E, Babar A, Choudhary M, Kutner M, Pyrsopoulos N. Acetaminophen-induced Hepatotoxicity: A Comprehensive Update. J Clin Transl Hepatol. 2016;4(2):131-42.

Case 6.3

Acute Pancreatitis

COMPETENCY

❖ **BC14.19:** Explain the basis and rationale of Biochemical tests done and interpretation of laboratory results in pancreatitis

Case Scenario

A 28-year-old male came to emergency department with complaints of severe abdominal pain in the upper abdomen since last 4 to 6 hours, pain is also radiating to the back and was not relieved by analgesics. He occasionally consumes alcohol. He revealed the history of similar type of symptoms, few days back. He also said that he consumed alcohol and heavy oily food last night.

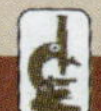

Laboratory Findings Reveal

- Serum lipase—300 IU/L (0–160 IU/L)
- Serum amylase—250 IU/L (40–140 IU/L)
- Serum ALT—70 IU/L (10–40 IU/L)
- Serum AST—60 IU/L (8–20 IU/L)

QUESTIONS

Q.1. What is the probable diagnosis? Explain its biochemical basis.

Q.2. What other biochemical derangements could be found?

Q.3. What should be the treatment plan for the case?

ANSWERS

A.1. Probable diagnosis is acute pancreatitis. Two most common causes of the condition:

1. Biliary duct obstruction (≈40%)
2. Alcohol abuse (≈35%).

Other causes may be:

3. Trauma
4. Hyperlipidemia
5. Drugs
6. Autoimmune
7. Idiopathic

Above case seems to be due to excess alcohol intake. There are two ways for catabolism of alcohol in pancreas—oxidative and non-oxidative. Later one is dominating and results in formation of fatty acid ethyl esters (FAEEs). Accumulation of these products causes pancreatic acinar cell damage.

Damage to pancreatic acinar cell, causes release of enzymes amylase and lipase. Lipase is more specific than amylase as it is elevated within 4–8 hours of pain onset and remain elevated for 7–10 days. Whereas amylase rises within 6 hours of pain onset and normalizes in blood by 3–5 days. So for diagnosing acute pancreatitis, either in early and late stages, lipase has a better degree of sensitivity and specificity to diagnose the disease. Lipase is more specific too as it is mainly secreted from pancreas. Amylase may also increase in other conditions like renal failure, mumps parotitis, esophageal perforation.

A.2. Parameters for liver function tests may be altered:
- Increase ALT, AST, ALP and bilirubin and decrease serum albumin.
- Blood sugar may be deranged due to insulin producing β-cell dysfunction.
- Serum calcium may be decreased due to hypoalbuminemia.

A.3. Acute pancreatitis can be manage in hospital setup only because of close monitoring of vital signs and symptoms of disease is essential. Other supportive measures are:
- Analgesic for pain
- Nil by mouth (NBM), IV fluids to manage the dehydration
- Antibiotic prophylaxis to reduce the mortality.

In most of the cases (≈90%) symptoms subsides spontaneously within 3 to 7 days. Once the condition is under control, underlying cause need to be focused as like gallstones, chronic alcoholism.

BIBLIOGRAPHY

1. Chatila AT, Bilal M, Guturu P. Evaluation and management of acute pancreatitis. World J Clin Cases. 2019;7(9):1006-1020.
2. Gapp J, Chandra S. Acute Pancreatitis. [Updated 2022 Jun 21]. In: StatPearls [Internet]. Treasure Island (FL): StatPearls Publishing; 2022. Available from: https://www.ncbi.nlm.nih.gov/books/NBK482468.

Case 6.4

Acute Hepatitis

COMPETENCY

❖ **BC2.4:** Describe and discuss the clinical utility of various serum enzymes in laboratory and their use as markers of various pathological conditions

Integration with Medicine

❖ **GM5.3:** Describe and discuss the epidemiology, microbiology, Immunology and clinical evolution of infective (viral) hepatitis

Case Scenario

A 25-year-old male suffered from loss of appetite, nausea, fever and pain in right hypochondrium since last two days. He revealed the history of eating outside food 3 days back. On examination, it was found that the liver was palpable and tender. Color of random urine was yellow **(Table 6.4.1)**.

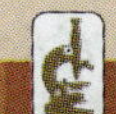

Laboratory Findings Reveal

- Serum total bilirubin: 6.0 mg/dL (0.2–1.2 mg/dL)
- Serum direct bilirubin: 3.0 mg/dL (0–0.2 mg/dL)
- Serum indirect bilirubin: 3.0 mg/dL (0.2–0.7 mg/dL)
- ALT: 1550 IU/L (10–40 IU/L)
- AST: 935 IU/L (8–20 IU/L)
- ALP: 215 IU/L (40–130 IU/L)
- Serum total protein: 7.0 g/dL (6–8 g/dL)
- Serum albumin: 4.2 g/dL (3.5–5 g/dL)

Table 6.4.1: Clinical presentation of hepatitis.

Acute	*Chronic*
◆ Fever ◆ Malaise ◆ Myalgia and arthralgia ◆ Nausea or vomiting ◆ Loss of appetite ◆ Abdominal pain ◆ Dark urine ◆ Clay-colored stool ◆ Jaundice	◆ Fatigue ◆ Weight loss ◆ Peripheral edema ◆ Ascites

QUESTIONS

Q.1. What is the probable diagnosis? What can be the causes for the above condition?

Q.2. Explain the biochemical basis for laboratory findings. Why the level of ALT is more than AST?

Q.3. What treatment should be advised to the patient?

ANSWERS

A.1. Probable diagnosis is acute hepatitis. Hepatitis is the infection of hepatocytes. Depending upon the etiology hepatitis may be:

- Viral hepatitis
- Bacterial hepatitis
- Alcoholic hepatitis
- Drugs or toxins induced hepatitis
- Ischemic hepatitis.

A.2. Acute inflammation of the hepatocytes increases the permeability of hepatocytes, causes release of enzymes ALT and AST from the hepatocytes. As the AST has both cytoplasmic and mitochondrial fractions, so its level is comparatively less than ALT in acute condition. Infected hepatocytes are not being able to uptake and conjugate the unconjugated bilirubin effectively, that is why the level of unconjugated bilirubin increases and at the same time inflammation lead to swelling of the cells, causes intrahepatic biliary obstruction, so whatever bilirubin is conjugated, is not able to excrete out through bile results in rise in conjugated bilirubin. In acute liver disease, albumin levels remain unchanged as the half-life of albumin is about three weeks.

A.3. Management of hepatitis patient is mainly supportive in nature:

- Maintain the hydration by drinking enough fluids to prevent dehydration
- Approx 99% recovery occurs spontaneously, anti-viral therapy is needed in rare condition of severe acute hepatitis.

BIBLIOGRAPHY

1. Mehta P, Reddivari AKR. Hepatitis. [Updated 2022 Sep 30]. In: StatPearls [Internet]. Treasure Island (FL): StatPearls Publishing; 2022. Available from: https://www.ncbi.nlm.nih.gov/books/NBK554549/
2. Schaefer TJ, John S. Acute Hepatitis. [Updated 2022 Jul 18]. In: StatPearls [Internet]. Treasure Island (FL): StatPearls Publishing; 2022. Available from: https://www.ncbi.nlm.nih.gov/books/NBK551570/

Case 6.5

Methanol Poisoning

COMPETENCY

- **BC2.3:** Describe and discuss enzyme Inhibition and role of enzymes or drugs as Inhibitors, and enzymes as therapeutic agents

Integration with Medicine

- **GM22.4:** Enumerate the commonly observed drug overdose in your area and describe their toxicology, clinical features, prognosis and approach to therapy

Case Scenario

A 56-year-old male brought to hospital in an unconscious state. His body temperature was 36°C, heart beat 118 beats/minutes, respiration rate 26, pupils were reactive to light. Family members revealed the history of consumption of liquor from local vendor. Following 5 to 6 hours, he develops stunning of speech and blurring of vision and become unconscious.

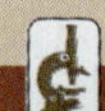

Laboratory Findings Reveal

- pH: 7.05 (7.35–7.45)
- Serum HCO_3: 7.9 µmol/L (22–26 µmol/L)
- Serum Na: 140 mEq/L (136–145 mEq/L/L)
- Serum K: 4.27 mEq/L (3.5–5 mEq/L/L)
- Serum Cl: 106 mEq/L (96–106 mEq/L/L)
- Serum albumin: 4.2 g/dL (3.5–5 g/dL)

QUESTIONS

Q.1. Identify the case. Explain the biochemical basis for the condition.

Q.2. Enlist the other deferential diagnosis of this condition.

Q.3. What treatment should be advised to the patient?

ANSWERS

A.1. Probable diagnosis is methanol poisoning.

Methanol is readily absorbed through intestine and reaches to circulation within 10 minutes. It is metabolized in liver to form formaldehyde being highly toxic causes damage to retinal cells and formic acid results in severe metabolic acidosis and its consequences **(Fig. 6.5.1)**.

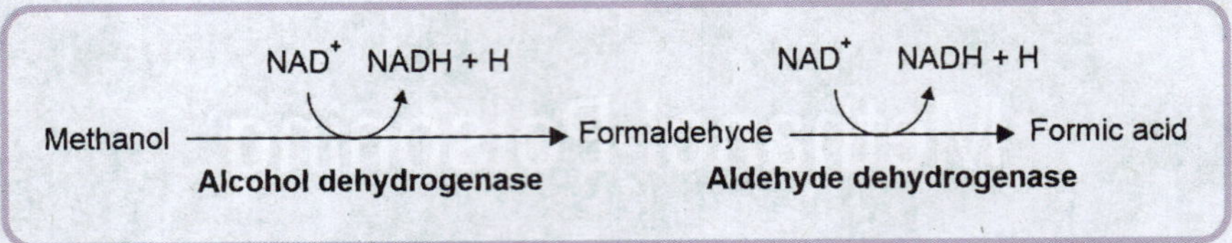

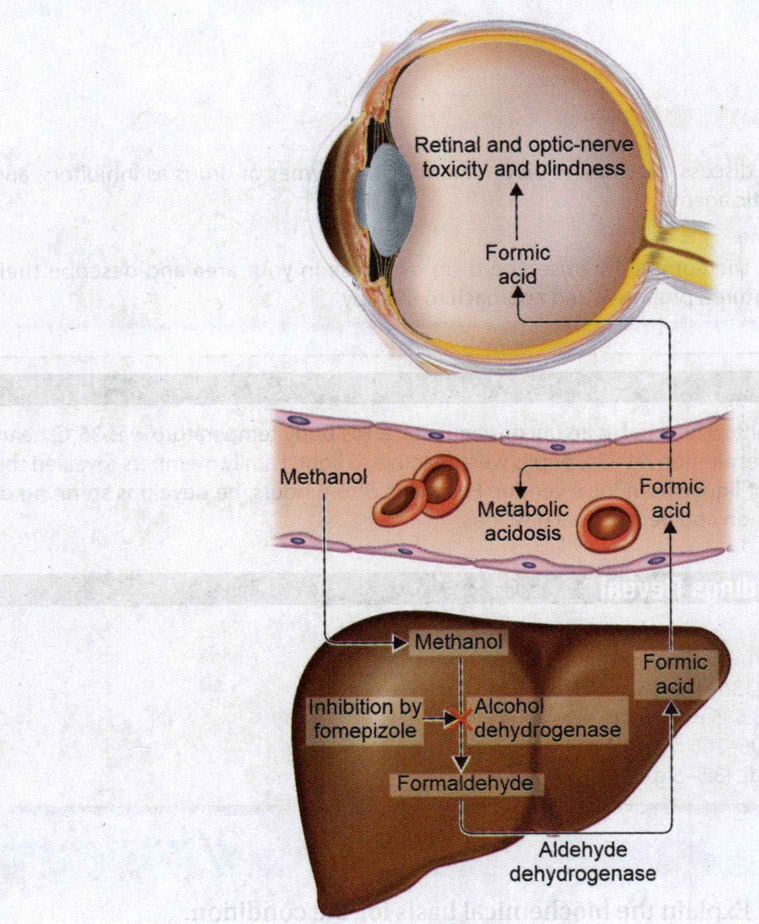

Fig. 6.5.1: Pathogenesis of alcohol toxicity.

A.2. Patients is having high anion gap metabolic acidosis other condition which can result in high anion gap metabolic acidosis:

- Diabetic ketoacidosis
- Ethyl glycol
- Isoniazid
- Lactate
- Methanol

- Propylene glycol
- Salicylates
- Uremia

A.3. Along with other corrective measures for metabolic acidosis, ethyl alcohol is given as antidote for treatment. This is the competitive inhibitor of alcohol dehydrogenase and its metabolic product acetaldehyde and acetic acid are less toxic. Fomepizole is used as antidote for methanol as it inhibits the enzyme alcohol dehydrogenase.

BIBLIOGRAPHY

1. Brubaker RH, Vashisht R, Meseeha M. High Anion Gap Metabolic Acidosis. [Updated 2022 Aug 8]. In: StatPearls [Internet]. Treasure Island (FL): StatPearls Publishing; 2022. Available from: https://www.ncbi.nlm.nih.gov/books/NBK448090/
2. Jung YC, Namkoong K. Alcohol: intoxication and poisoning-diagnosis and treatment. Handb Clin Neurol. 2014;125:115-21.
3. LaHood AJ, Kok SJ. Ethanol Toxicity. [Updated 2022 Mar 18]. In: StatPearls [Internet]. Treasure Island (FL): StatPearls Publishing; 2022. Available from: https://www.ncbi.nlm.nih.gov/books/NBK557381/

GIVE REASONS WHY

Q.1. Some enzymes exist as isoenzymes.

Ans. Isoenzymes are physical distinct form of the same enzyme. It means they catalyze same reaction but have different physical properties. They have same domain but the number and sequence of amino acids can be different in other regions in the structure. For such enzymes genes are different.

Types of isoenzymes

True isoenzyme: Produce from different gene (salivary and pancreatic amylase).

Allozymes: These genes can be present on same locus, but may have different alleles (different form of G6PD by the same locus on X-chromosomes, when isoenzymes due to variation at a single locus occur with appreciable frequency (more than 1% of total population) it is known as polymorphism.

Isoforms: When difference in enzyme occurs due to post-translational modification (addition of sialic acid in alkaline phosphate).

Q.2. Methotrexate is used as an anticancer drug.

Ans. Methotrexate competitively inhibits the enzyme folate reductase. This drug is a structural analogue of folic acid. **Folate reductase** is required to synthesize active form of folic acid which is further needed for DNA synthesis and cell replication.

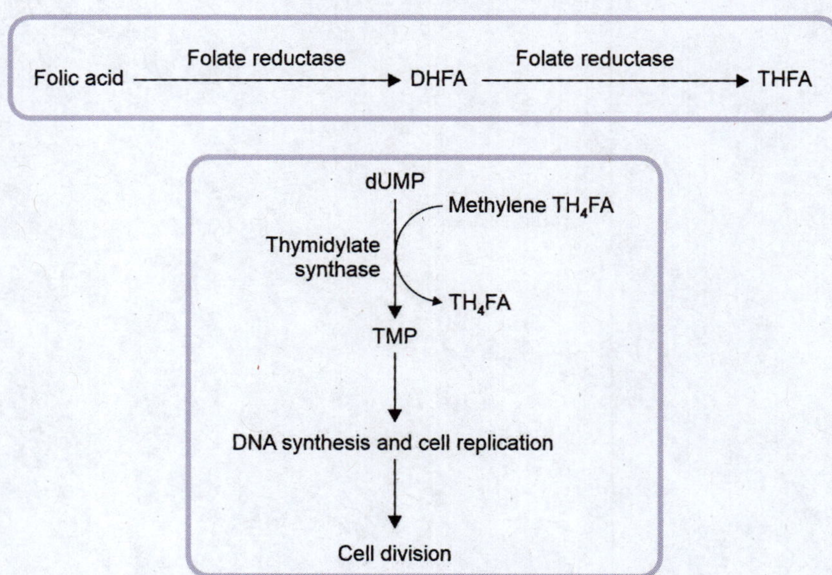

Q.3. Sulfa drugs have bacteriostatic effect.

Ans. Bacterial cells cannot use the host folic acid for their own (folic acid is required for cell division). So they have to synthesize their own folic acid by combining PABA with pteroyl glutamic acid with the help of enzyme pteroid synthetase. Sulfa drugs are structural analogue of PABA and competitively inhibit pteroid synthetase. So reduces synthesis of folic acid in bacteria, reduces cell division known as bacteriostatic drugs.

Q.4. Dicumarol used as anticoagulant drug.

Ans. Dicumarol inhibits the enzyme vitamin-K epoxide reductase. This is one of the enzymes required to regenerate active form of vitamin K (reduced form). This reduced form is essential for gamma carboxylation of clotting factors, these activated clotting factors helps in blood coagulation.

Q.5. Statin drugs are used to lower blood cholesterol.

Ans. Statin drugs are competitive inhibitor for the enzyme HMG-CoA reductase which regulates the **committed step** of cholesterol synthesis.

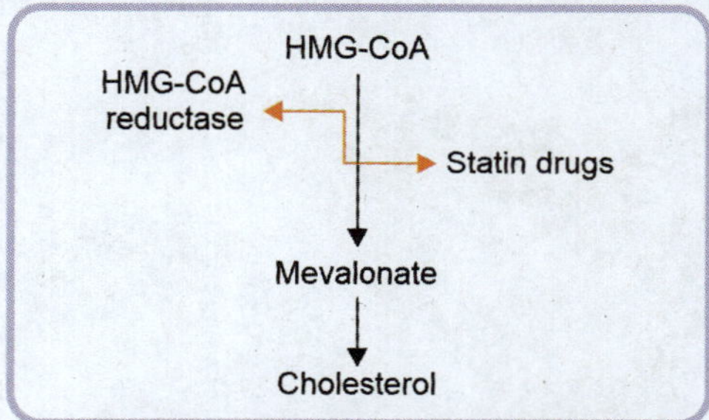

Q.6. Enzymes shows maximum activity at optimum pH.

Ans. Optimum pH far an enzyme is that pH, where enzyme activity is maximum. At this pH or H^+ concentration enzymes are ionized in such a way that favors formation of maximum (ES) complex.

Q.7. Urokinase or streptokinase is given in treatment of myocardial infarction.

Ans. When myocardial infarction results due to thrombosis or thrombus formation in coronary artery, urokinase/streptokinase are helpful as these enzymes are plasminogen activators (PA) which covert plasminogen into plasmin. Plasmin is responsible for degradation of fibrin and dissolution of fibrin clot.

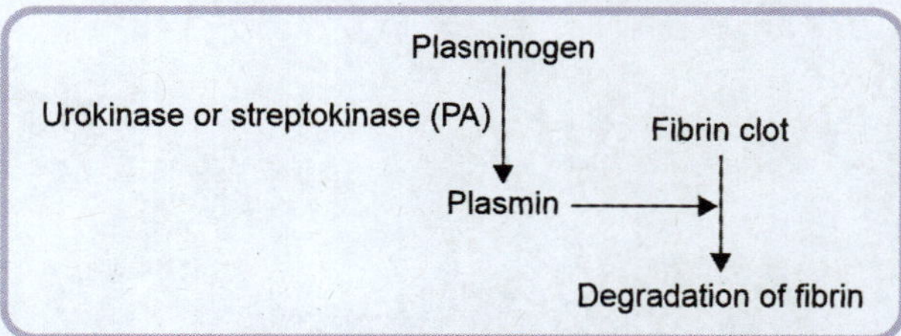

Q.8. Asparaginase is given in treatment of cancer.

Ans. Cancer cells are not being able to synthesize their own asparagine and it can be provided to them only through blood supply. If asparaginase is injected it hydrolyses asparagine and so decrease its blood level and limit the availability of amino acid to cancer cells. In this way inhibit the growth and multiplication of cells.

Q.9. Scoline apnea (succinylcholine apnea) in patients with low cholinesterase activity.

Ans. Succinylcholine is given as muscle relaxant along with general anesthesia to the patients. Enzyme cholinesterase breaks succinylcholine within 2–4 minutes, but in patients with low activity of cholinesterase it takes hours to hydrolyze succinylcholine, that results in prolong muscle relaxation (specially respiratory muscles) causes scoline apnea.

Section

7 Heme and Hemoglobin Metabolism

- **Case 7.1:** Acute Intermittent Porphyria
- **Case 7.2:** Porphyria Cutanea Tarda
- **Case 7.3:** Obstructive Jaundice
- **Case 7.4:** Kernicterus
- **Case 7.5:** Hepatic Jaundice
- **Case 7.6:** Sickle Cell Anemia
- **Case 7.7:** Thalassemia

Give Reasons Why

Case 7.1

Acute Intermittent Porphyria

COMPETENCY

❖ **BC5.8:** Describe the structure and functions of haem in the body and describe the processes involved in its metabolism with emphasis on jaundice and describe porphyrin metabolism

Case Scenario

A 33-year-old woman presented in medicine outpatient department (OPD) with acute abdominal pain, vomiting and behavioral symptoms. She developed seizures, and rapidly progressive weakness and quadriplegia (paralysis of arms and legs). Patient had severe neuropathy resulting in significant disability.

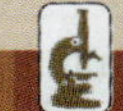

Laboratory Findings Reveal

- Serum Na^+—129 mmol/L (136–145 mmol/L)
- Serum K^+—3.8 mmol/L (3.5–5.0 mmol/L)
- Hemoglobin—7.0 g/dL (12–16 g/dL)
- Liver and pancreatic function test—within normal levels
- CSF analysis—within normal levels
- Urine analysis—porphobilinogen present in urine
- Color—fluorescent pink

QUESTIONS

Q.1. What is the most probable diagnosis and cause of this clinical condition?

Q.2. Explain the biochemical basis of such clinical presentation. Why this clinical condition is more prevalent in females?

Q.3. Enumerate other differential diagnosis of such a clinical presentation, how you confirm your diagnosis.

Q.4. What is the line of management in this patient?

ANSWERS

A.1. Patients is most probably suffering from acute intermittent porphyria. Porphyria's are group of metabolic disorders due to inherited deficiency of enzymes responsible for heme synthesis Clinical presentation of acute intermittent porphyria is summarized in **Table 7.1.1**. Porphyria can be classified as acute (neurological) and nonacute (cutaneous) **(Table 7.1.2)**. The term "acute porphyria" is used to describe porphyria's that can be associated with sudden attacks of pain and other neurological symptoms. Porphyria's can be classified into the "hepatic" and "erythropoietic" types.

Table 7.1.1: Clinical presentation of acute intermittent porphyria.
• **Peripheral nervous system:** Numbness, fatigue, tiredness, respiratory paralysis, sensory loss, limb weakness
• **Central nervous system:** Confusion, anxiety, depression, seizures, insomnia, hallucinations
• **Autonomic nervous system:** Unexplained abdominal pain, pain in back and chest, nausea and vomiting
• **Gastrointestinal symptoms:** Constipation and diarrhea
• **Cardiovascular symptoms:** High blood pressure, increased heart rate
• **Other nonspecific symptoms:** Dark colored urine, low blood sodium

Table 7.1.2: Types of porphyria.

Type	*Name of porphyria*	*Tissue*	*Inheritance*
Acute porphyria (neurological porphyria)	ALAD deficiency porphyria	Liver	Autosomal recessive
	Acute intermittent porphyria	Liver	Autosomal dominant
	Hereditary coproporphyria (photosensitivity is present)	Liver	Autosomal dominant
	Variegate porphyria (photosensitivity is present)	Liver	Autosomal dominant
Non-acute porphyrias (cutaneous porphyria)	Porphyria cutanea tarda	Liver	Autosomal dominant
	Erythropoietic protoporphyria	Erythroid cells and liver	Autosomal dominant
	Congenital erythropoietic porphyria	Erythroid cells	Autosomal recessive
Secondary prophyria	Lead poisoning Iron deficiency Coproporphyrinuria		

Acute intermittent porphyria (AIP) autosomal dominant metabolic disorder. It is most common porphyria with prevalence of 1:10,000 that is characterized by partial deficiency of the enzyme hydroxymethylbilane synthase (also known as porphobilinogen deaminase). This enzyme deficiency is caused by a mutation in the HMBS gene. Though, enzyme deficiency itself is not sufficient to produce symptoms, additional factors such as hormonal changes associated with puberty, the use of certain prescribed or recreational drugs, excess alcohol consumption, infections, and fasting or dietary changes are required to trigger the appearance of symptoms.

A.2. Biochemical basis of clinical presentation of acute intermittent porphyria.

There is an inherited deficiency of enzyme hydroxymethylbilane synthase (porphobilinogen deaminase) of heme synthesis. This enzyme deficiency can result in the accumulation of porphyrin precursors in the body. Accumulation of the porphyrin precursors, porphobilinogen, and aminolevulinic acid (ALA) leads to neurological damages.

Though the inheritance of this clinical disorder is autosomal, but it is more prevalent is female patients because female hormones especially progesterone has stimulatory effect on ALA synthase and that is why severity of disease is less in postmenopausal and prepubertal patients compare to patients of reproductive age group.

Metabolic reactions of heme synthesis are summarized in **Figure 7.1.1**.

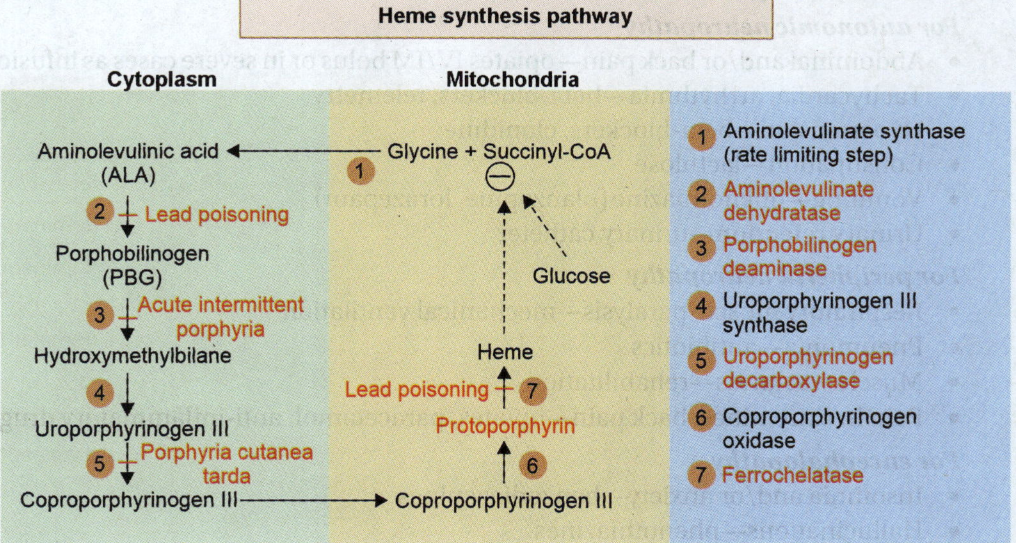

Fig. 7.1.1: Heme synthesis.

A.3. A diagnosis of AIP can be difficult because most symptoms are nonspecific and occur episodically. Other disorders which can be present with similar presentations are:

- Three other forms of porphyria specifically variegate porphyria, hereditary coproporphyria, and ALA-dehydratase deficiency porphyria
- Guillain-Barré syndrome (GBS)
- Tyrosinemia type I
- Lead toxicity.

Confirmation of diagnosis can be done with:

- The clinical criteria of an acute attack include the paroxysmal nature of the symptoms with abdominal or back pain associated with one or more signs of autonomic dysfunction, hyponatremia, muscle weakness, or mental symptoms.

- Biochemical criteria of an acute attack include more than a five-fold increase of urinary porphobilinogen (PBG) excretion, which can be detected by a simple Watson-Schwartz or Hoesch qualitative test.

A.4. Management of acute intermittent porphyria

Management primarily focused on to treat symptoms, prevent complications and to suppress heme synthesis in the liver with hematin, which reduces the production of porphyrin precursors.

Specific therapy

- Heme preparations (3–4 mg/kg/d for 3–4 consequent days)
- Glucose and other fluid infusions and follow-up of electrolytes, carbohydrate rich food

Supportive therapy

For autonomic neuropathy

- Abdominal and/or back pain—opiates IV/IM bolus or in severe cases as infusion
- Tachycardia, arrhythmia—beta-blockers, telemetry
- Hypertension—beta-blockers, clonidine
- Constipation—lactulose
- Vomiting—phenothiazine (olanzapine, lorazepam)
- Urinary retention—urinary catheter

For peripheral neuropathy

- Respiratory muscle paralysis—mechanical ventilation
- Pneumonia—antibiotics
- Muscle weakness—rehabilitation
- Pain in extremities, back pain—opiates, paracetamol, anti-inflammatory drugs

For encephalopathy

- Insomnia and/or anxiety—benzodiazepines
- Hallucinations—phenothiazines
- Convulsions—correction of hyponatremia and hypertension, diazepam

For metabolic changes

- Hyponatremia—correct water and electrolyte imbalance
- Acute renal failure—hemodialysis
- Liver injury—monitoring of SGOT/SGPT
- Dark urine—monitoring of urinary porphobilinogen (PBG) and urinary alpha levulinic acid (ALA)

BIBLIOGRAPHY

1. https://rarediseases.org/rare-diseases/acute-intermittent-porphyria/
2. Pischik E, Kauppinen R. An update of clinical management of acute intermittent porphyria. Appl Clin Genet. 2015;8:201-14.

Case 7.2

Porphyria Cutanea Tarda

COMPETENCY

❖ **BC5.8:** Describe the structure and functions of haem in the body and describe the processes involved in its metabolism with emphasis on jaundice and describe porphyrin metabolism

Case Scenario

A 59-year-old man presented dark red colored urine and also complain of fatigue, loss of energy, hyper- pigmented scar on his hands and face after exposure to sun which was started with blister and healed leaving a scar. His medical history and family history were both unremarkable. He is a chronic smoker and nonvegetarian and declared that his complaints exaggerated after consuming nonvegetarian diet.

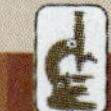

Laboratory Findings Reveal

- Serum aspartate aminotransferase (AST): 125 U/L (8–20)
- Serum alanine aminotransferase (ALT): 89 U/L (10–40)
- Serum lactate dehydrogenase (LDH): 268 (0–248)
- Serum alkaline phosphatase (ALP): 123 U/L (40–130)
- Serum ferritin: 503 ng/mL (15–200)
- Urine—dark red colored and turbid
- Hepatitis C, hepatitis B, and HIV tests were negative
- Autoimmune screening was negative
- 24-hour urine analysis shows increased porphyrin levels

QUESTIONS

Q.1. What is the most probable diagnosis and cause of this clinical condition?

Q.2. Explain the biochemical basis of such clinical presentation.

Q.3. Enumerate other differential diagnosis of such a clinical presentation, how you confirm your diagnosis?

Q.4. What is the line of management in this patient?

ANSWERS

A.1. Patient is suffering from porphyria cutanea tarda (PCT). PCT the second most common porphyria, is the result of a deficiency of the enzyme uroporphyrinogen decarboxylase (UROD). The hallmark of this disorder is photosensitivity, factors that can trigger the clinical manifestations of PCT are as follows:

- Alcohol: 80% to 90% of patients with PCT manifestations have a history of heavy alcohol consumption
- Hepatitis C virus (HCV)
- Estrogen
- HIV
- Hemochromatosis
- Smoking

A.2. Biochemical basis of clinical presentation

Accumulation of porphyrins in different organs, especially the liver and skin, leads to the clinical manifestations seen in patients. These porphyrins spills into the bloodstream and when interacts with light, especially blue light, with a wavelength of 410 nm, initially excites and subsequently go back to their original ground state after releasing energy. This energy is transferred to molecular oxygen and creates 'singlet-excited oxygen' which is implicated in oxidizing several essential biological compounds like lipids, proteins, and causes peroxidation of cell membrane lipids, disintegrates cell membrane, and eventually leads to cell death.

A.3. Differential diagnosis of above clinical condition can be:

- Hereditary coproporphyria
- Variegate porphyria
- Congenital erythropoietic porphyria
- Blistering skin diseases, such as epidermolysis bullosa, polymorphous light eruptions

Porphyrin elevation is also seen in liver disease, advanced renal disease, and other porphyrias. However, they will not show the typical cutaneous manifestations seen in patients with PCT.

A.4. Management of PCT includes avoidance of precipitating and susceptibility factors. As this is a photosensitive skin condition, sunlight avoidance is the crucial. Sunscreen containing titanium dioxide or zinc oxide, protective clothing is helpful in protecting the skin from harmful sunlight rays. Alcohol, smoking, excess iron intake, and estrogen therapy should be avoided strictly.

The mainstay therapies of PCT are phlebotomy and hydroxychloroquine. Iron chelation therapy is also useful alternative.

BIBLIOGRAPHY

1. Shah A, Bhatt H. Cutanea tarda porphyria. [Updated 2022 May 13]. In: StatPearls [Internet]. Treasure Island (FL): StatPearls Publishing; 2022.
2. Usta Atmaca H, Akbas F. Porphyria cutanea tarda: A case report. J Med Case Reports. 2019;13:17.

Case 7.3

Obstructive Jaundice

COMPETENCY

- ❖ **BC14.19:** Explain the basis and rationale of biochemical tests done and interpretation of laboratory results in Jaundice

Integration with Medicine

- ❖ **GM5.1:** Describe and discuss the physiologic and biochemical basis of hyperbilirubinemia

Integration with Pathology

- ❖ **PA24.1:** Describe Bilirubin metabolism, enumerate the etiology and pathogenesis of jaundice, distinguish between direct and indirect hyperbilirubinemia

Case Scenario

A 40-year-old male came to clinic with complain of mild epigastric pain with fever. Also, there was a history of vomiting and clay color stools after eating fatty food. On examination, there was mild hepatomegaly and he was advised abdominal ultrasound and liver function test (LFT).

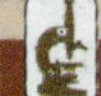

Laboratory Findings Reveal

- Serum total bilirubin: 10 mg/dL
- Serum direct bilirubin: 8.5 mg/dL
- Serum indirect bilirubin: 1.5 mg/dL
- Serum alkaline phosphatase: 320 IU/L
- Serum AST: 42 IU/L
- Serum ALT: 35 IU/L
- Urine bile salt: Present
- Urine bile pigment: Present
- Urine urobilinogen: Absent
- Ultrasound showed presence of gallstones

QUESTIONS

Q.1. What is your probable diagnosis? What can be the other causes for such clinical presentation?

Q.2. Explain the presence of bile salt and bile pigment in the urine sample, name of the test to detect presence of bile salt and bile pigment in urine.

Q.3. What laboratory investigations are helpful in confirmation of clinical condition?

Q.4. What is the line of management in this clinical condition?

ANSWERS

A.1. Patient most probably suffering from obstructive jaundice. Other reasons could be:

- Intrahepatic biliary obstruction after followed by chronic hepatitis or due to biliary stones
- Pancreatic carcinoma
- Biliary stricture
- Gallstones
- Severe inflammation of liver
- Hepatoma

Clinical presentation of obstructive jaundice is summarized in **Table 7.3.1**.

Table 7.3.1: Clinical presentation of obstructive jaundice.
• Jaundice, dark urine, clay color stool
• Pruritus
• Weight loss, nausea, vomiting
• Right upper abdominal pain
• Charcot's triad (upper abdominal pain, fever and jaundice)
• Reynold's pentad (upper abdominal pain, fever and jaundice, confusion and hypotension)

A.2. Obstruction in the bile duct restricts the excretion of bile from liver to intestine, so there will be absence of bile in feces as well as the urobilinogen in urine. Bile regurgitates in the circulation and results in an increase in conjugated (direct) bilirubin and bile salts in blood and as it is water-soluble it excretes out in urine also. Presence of bile salt and bile pigment can be easily checked by Hay's sulfur powder test (bile salt) and Fouchet's test (bile pigment).

A.3. There are various laboratory tests which can be helpful to confirm diagnosis of patient.

Blood Tests

- Complete blood count (CBC)
- Comprehensive metabolic profile (CMP)
- Fractionated bilirubin
- Alkaline phosphatase and fractionation
- Gamma-glutamyl transferase (GGT)
- Viral hepatitis serology
- Antimitochondrial antibody levels
- Antinuclear antibody
- Coagulation studies
- Tumor markers (CA19-9, CEA, AFP)

Urine Test

Urine bilirubin.

Stool Test

Occult blood to rule out GI malignancy.

Radiological and Endoscopic Tests

1. **Abdominal ultrasound with Doppler**—it is a good test to evaluate for gallstones, dilations of extrahepatic bile ducts, and assessing for patency of blood vessels using Doppler.
2. **Abdominal CT scan**—it can be useful in pancreatic head lesions, liver lesions.
3. **Nuclear medicine scans** like the HIDA scan can assess for cystic duct obstruction.
4. **MRCP (magnetic resonance cholangiopancreatography)**—it is useful in detection of intra and extrahepatic bile duct abnormalities.
5. **Invasive diagnostic and therapeutic endoscopic ultrasound (EUS)** with needle aspiration and endoscopic retrograde cholangiopancreatography (ERCP) with biopsies.

A.4. Management of patient with biliary obstruction include:

Initial management for acute cholangitis requires admission to hospital for IVF resuscitation and electrolyte replacement, pain control and antibiotics. Treatment for biliary obstruction depends on the cause but likely will be either surgical or nonsurgical.

Nonsurgical may include stabilization and pain control along with medications to help dissolve gallstones causing an obstruction.

Surgical may include cholecystectomy to remove the gallbladder if the cause is gallstones along with ERCP with sphincterotomy to remove gallstones from the biliary tract causing an obstruction.

BIBLIOGRAPHY

1. Coucke EM, Akbar H, Kahloon A, et al. Biliary obstruction. [Updated 2022 Sep 26]. In: StatPearls [Internet]. Treasure Island (FL): StatPearls Publishing; 2022 Jan-. Available from: https://www.ncbi.nlm. nih.gov/books/NBK539698/
2. Taylor T, Wheatley M, Gupta N, Nusbaum J. Jaundice in the emergency department: Meeting the challenges of diagnosis and treatment [digest]. Emerg Med Pract. 2018;20(Suppl 4):1-2.

Case 7.4

Kernicterus

COMPETENCY

❖ **BC14.19:** Explain the basis and rationale of biochemical tests done and interpretation of laboratory results in Jaundice

Integration with Medicine

❖ **GM5.1:** Describe and discuss the physiologic and biochemical basis of hyperbilirubinemia

Integration with Pathology

❖ **PA24.1:** Describe Bilirubin metabolism, enumerate the etiology and pathogenesis of jaundice, distinguish between direct and indirect hyperbilirubinemia

Case Scenario

A 5-day-old infant presented with increasing icterus, poor suck and high pitched cry. On examination he found drowsy, lethargic with reduced muscles tone. There was a history of jaundice in elder sibling (blood group not known).

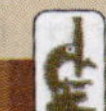

Laboratory Findings Reveal

- Blood glucose—80 mg/dL (70–110 mg/dL)
- Hemoglobin Levels—6 g/dL (>16 g/dL)
- Serum bilirubin—27 mg/dL (<20 mg/dL in first 72 hours)
- Newborn blood group A^+
- Mother blood group O^+
- Mother anti-A antibodies detected with high titer

QUESTIONS

Q.1. What is the most probable diagnosis and causes of such clinical condition?

Q.2. What is the biochemical basis of such clinical presentation?

Q.3. What are the other investigations required to confirm your diagnosis?

Q.4. What is the line of management?

ANSWERS

A.1. Child is suffering from kernicterus (bilirubin encephalopathy). Hyperbilirubinemia is one of the most common neonatal disorders. Delayed diagnosis and treatment of the pathologic and progressive indirect hyperbilirubinemia lead to neurological deficits, defined as bilirubin induced encephalopathy. Clinical presentation of bilirubin encephalopathy (kernicterus) is summarized in **Figure 7.4.1.**

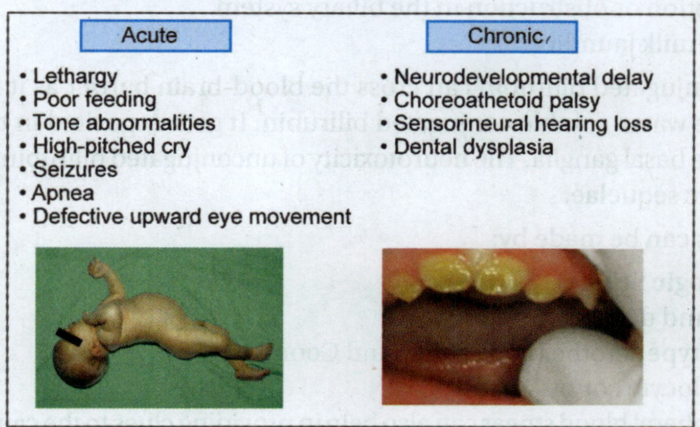

Fig. 7.4.1: Clinical presentation of bilirubin encephalopathy (kernicterus).

Conditions which can lead to kernicterus may be:

a. Blood group incompatibility between newborn and mother
b. Glucose-6-phosphate dehydrogenase (G6PD) deficiency
c. Premature birth, sepsis, meningitis
d. Drugs like sulfonamides, cotrimoxazole

A.2. Biochemical basis of kernicterus

Kernicterus occurs when the unconjugated bilirubin (indirect bilirubin) levels cross 25 mg/dL in the blood from any event leading to decreased elimination and increased production of bilirubin.

Increased production of bilirubin resulting from:

1. **Polycythemia**—increased number of red blood cells leads to an increase in their turnover.
2. **Hemolysis**—varied causes such as erythroblastosis fetalis, ABO blood group incompatibility as happened in above case, hemolytic disease of the newborn, and abnormalities of the red cell itself such as hereditary spherocytosis, elliptocytosis, G6PD deficiency, pyruvate kinase deficiency; and hemoglobinopathies, such as alpha and beta-thalassemia.
3. **Birth injuries**—cephalohematoma, subgaleal hemorrhage, or peripheral ecchymosis from birth trauma.

Causes of decreased excretion are:

1. **Hypoalbuminemia**—as the unconjugated bilirubin is lipid-soluble, it is normally bound to albumin, a decrease in the albumin level leads to an increase in free unconjugated bilirubin level.
2. **Hereditary bilirubin conjugation defects**—Crigler-Najjar syndrome and Gilbert syndrome are due to the deficiency of the enzyme uridine 5'-diphosphate-glucuronosyltransferase (UDPGT), which conjugates the bilirubin in the liver cells.
3. Disruption or obstruction in the biliary system.
4. Breast milk jaundice.

The unconjugated bilirubin can cross the blood-brain barrier as it is lipid-soluble, unlike the water-soluble conjugated bilirubin. It gets deposited in the brain tissue, mainly the basal ganglia. The neurotoxicity of unconjugated bilirubin leads to various neurologic sequelae.

A.3. Diagnosis can be made by:

Hematologic Studies

- Total and direct bilirubin
- Blood type (mother and infant) and Coombs test
- Reticulocyte count
- A peripheral blood smear can also help in providing clues to the cause of hemolysis.
- Complete blood count
- Serum electrolytes.

A.4. The main objective of the management of kernicterus is to prevent neurotoxicity by reducing bilirubin levels. The three mainstays of therapy to prevent and treat hyperbilirubinemia are:

a. **Exchange transfusion therapy:** Serum bilirubin levels more than 25–30 mg/dL are usually treated with an exchange transfusion.

b. **Phototherapy:** Phototherapy use of light to convert insoluble bilirubin molecules in the body into water-soluble isomers that can be excreted by the body, it is indicated when:
   - Equal or more than 15 mg/dL in infants 25–48 hours old
   - Equal or more than 18 mg/dL in infants 49–72 hours old
   - Equal or more than 20 mg/dL in infants older than 72 hours

c. **Intravenous immunoglobulins (IVIG):** This is indicated in immunologically mediated hemolytic conditions.

BIBLIOGRAPHY

1. Karimzadeh P, Fallahi M, Kazemian M, et al. Bilirubin induced encephalopathy. Iranian Journal of Child Neurology. 2020;14(1):7-19.
2. Reddy DK, Pandey S. Kernicterus. In: StatPearls [Internet]. Treasure Island (FL): StatPearls Publishing. 2022.
3. Springer SC. Kernicterus. New York: Medscape; 2014. [Cited 2018 Dec 10]. Available from: https://emedicine.medscape.com/

Case 7.5

Hepatic Jaundice

COMPETENCY

- ❖ **BC14.19:** Explain the basis and rationale of biochemical tests done and interpretation of laboratory results in Jaundice

Integration with Medicine

- ❖ **GM5.1:** Describe and discuss the physiologic and biochemical basis of hyperbilirubinemia

Integration with Pathology

- ❖ **PA24.1:** Describe Bilirubin metabolism, enumerate the etiology and pathogenesis of jaundice, distinguish between direct and indirect hyperbilirubinemia

Case Scenario

A 15-year-old boy admitted to emergency ward following episodes of fever, loss of appetite, nausea, and yellowish discoloration of eyes in last week. He also had an episode of occasional vomiting and pain in the right hypochondrium. On examination, he was looking pale and malnourished. Consultant asked for liver function test of the patient.

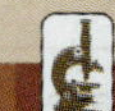

Laboratory Findings Reveal

LFT report of patient:

- Total bilirubin: 9 mg/dL
- Indirect bilirubin: 5.5 mg/dL
- Direct bilirubin: 3.5 mg/dL
- Serum AST: 560 IU/L
- Serum ALT: 620 IU/L
- Serum ALP: 45 IU/L

QUESTIONS

Q.1. What is your diagnosis in this patient? Justify the same, how can you made differential diagnosis with similar clinical presentation?

Q.2. Enlist various investigations comes under liver function test, add a comment on indication of liver function test.

Q.3. Outline the management and diet of the patient in brief.

ANSWERS

A.1. The patient is most probably suffering from acute hepatitis and hepatic jaundice. Because AST and ALT levels are markedly elevated and serum ALP levels are within the limit. Further the hyperbilirubinemia is of mixed type both direct and indirect bilirubin levels are elevated. Infection of hepatocytes results in decrease uptake of unconjugated bilirubin. High levels of direct bilirubin is due to intrahepatic obstruction of bile canaliculi caused by hepatocytic edema leading to intrahepatic stasis of bile. The direct bilirubin is therefore comes into circulation and manifests as hyperbilirubinemia.

Patient can have hemolytic or obstructive jaundice, lab results of different types of jaundice are summarized in **Table 7.5.1**.

Table 7.5.1: Lab results of different types of jaundice.

Test name	*Hemolytic jaundice*	*Hepatic jaundice*	*Obstructive jaundice*
Serum indirect bilirubin	Highly elevated	Elevated	Normal
Serum direct bilirubin	Normal	Elevated	Highly elevated
Serum aminotransferases (AST and ALT)	Normal	Highly elevated	Normal to moderately elevated
Serum alkaline phosphatase	Normal	Normal to moderately elevated (2–3 times than normal)	Highly elevated (5–8 times than normal)
Urine bile salts	Absent	++	+++
Urine bile pigments	Absent	+	+++
Urine urobilinogen	+++	Normal/+	Absent or in traces
Feces urobilins	++	Absent or in traces	Clay colored

A.2. Liver can be assessed based on its various functions. Following is the list of tests that can be done to check the status of liver:

Based on Excretory Functions

- Serum direct and total bilirubin
- Urine—bile salts and bile pigments

Based on Intermediary Metabolic Functions

- Prothrombin time
- Plasma amino acids levels

Based on Synthetic Role of Liver

- Serum albumin and globulin levels
- Assessment of various plasma proteins (e.g., ceruloplasmin, alpha-1 antitrypsin, etc.)

Based on Detoxification Functions

- Blood ammonia levels
- Hippuric acid synthesis test

Test to Check Liver Cell Damage

- Alkaline phosphatase (ALP)
- Aminotransferases (AST and ALT)
- Gamma-glutamyl transpeptidase (GGT)
- 5'-Nucleotidase

Indications of Liver Function Test

- To check, the presence of liver disease (such as hepatitis, cirrhosis, jaundice)
- To differentiate various liver diseases
- To distinguish types of jaundice
- To check the coagulation disorder
- To check the hepatotoxicity of various medicines (such as statins, antibiotics, acetaminophen, etc.)
- To monitor effectiveness of treatment

A.3. General supportive measures like symptomatic treatment and bed rest is advisable to reduce the load on liver low protein and low fat diet is advisable along with more fluids, which are rich in carbohydrates and electrolytes are advisable.

BIBLIOGRAPHY

1. Feuer G, Di Fonzo CJ. Intrahepatic cholestasis: a review of biochemical-pathological mechanisms. Drug Metabol Drug Interact. 1992;10(1-2):1-161.
2. Joseph A, Samant H. Jaundice. [Updated 2022 Aug 8]. In: StatPearls [Internet]. Treasure Island (FL): StatPearls Publishing; 2022. Available from: https://www.ncbi.nlm.nih.gov/books/NBK544252/

Case 7.6

Sickle Cell Anemia

COMPETENCY

- **BC5.9:** Describe the major types of Hemoglobin and its types, derivatives and variants found in the body and their physiological/pathological relevance

Integration with Pathology

- **PA16.2:** Describe the pathogenesis, features, hematologic indices and peripheral blood picture of sickle cell anemia and thalassemia

Case Scenario

A 7-year-old male child presented with mild pallor, icterus, abdominal and joint pains. On examination the child had mild splenomegaly. He had history of prior hospital admission for fever, anemia and jaundice. Family history of sibling death at 5 years of age due to fever and jaundice.

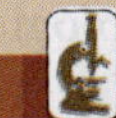

Laboratory Findings Reveal

- Hemoglobin—7.7 g/dL (12–16 g/dL)
- RBC—2.44 M/mm^3 (4.3–5.9 M/mm^3)
- Peripheral blood smear shows severe anisopoikilocytosis, microcytic hypochromic red cells, target cells, many boat cells, sickled RBCs, nucleated RBCs

QUESTIONS

Q.1. What is the most probable diagnosis of such a clinical condition?

Q.2. What investigation you require to confirm your diagnosis?

Q,3. What can be the other long-term complications in such a clinical disorder?

Q.4. What will be the line of management?

ANSWERS

A.1. Child is most probably suffering from sickle cell anemia.

Sickle cell disease (SCD) is the most common symptomatic hemoglobinopathy in the world, SCA is a monogenic disorder with an autosomal recessive inheritance. The parents are clinically asymptomatic and have normal blood counts.

Children may have a variable clinical course depending upon various genetic determinants, HbF levels and co-inheritance of other factors. Clinical presentation of sickle cell anemia is summarized in **Figure 7.6.1**.

- Anemia
- Episodes of pain—periodic episodes of extreme pain, called pain crises are major symptoms of sickle cell anemia
- Frequent infections, skin infection, leg ulcers
- Delayed growth or puberty
- Vision problems
- Renal disorders
- Hepatomegaly, autosplenectomy
- Gallbladder stones
- Priapism
- Bone marrow infarcts, arthritis

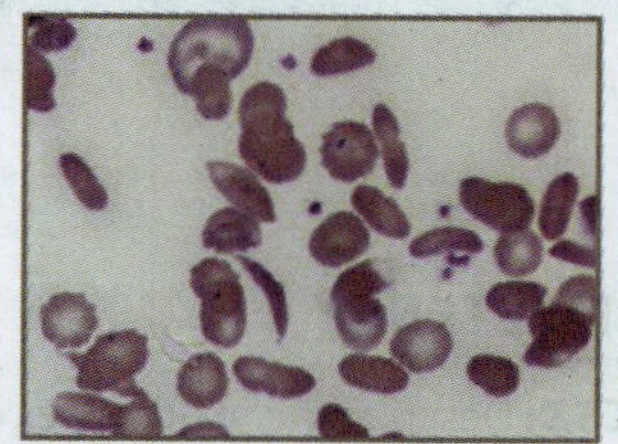

Fig. 7.6.1: Clinical presentation of sickle cell anemia.

A.2. Diagnosis mainly relies upon identification of HbS (by any of the following method):
- HPLC
- Hb electrophoresis
- Iso-electric focusing or sickling test

A.3. Patient of sickle cell anemia can have different complications including:
- Stroke
- Blindness
- Leg ulcers
- Gallstones
- Priapism
- Organ damage
- Splenic sequestration
- Deep vein thrombosis
- Acute chest syndrome
- Pulmonary hypertension

A.4. Treatment of sickle cell disease generally aims at relieving symptoms and preventing infections, sickle cell crises, and long-term complications. Stem cell transplant is the only potential cure available presently.

BIBLIOGRAPHY

1. Mangla A, Ehsan M, Agarwal N, et al. Sickle cell anemia. [Updated 2022 Nov 30]. In: StatPearls [Internet]. Treasure Island (FL): StatPearls Publishing; 2022.
2. Rees DC, Williams TN, Gladwin MT. Sickle-cell disease. Lancet. 2010;376(9757):2018-31.

Case 7.7

Thalassemia

COMPETENCY

- ❖ **BC5.9:** Describe the major types of Hemoglobin and its types, derivatives and variants found in the body and their physiological/pathological relevance

Integration with Pathology

- ❖ **PA16.2:** Describe the pathogenesis, features, hematologic indices and peripheral blood picture of sickle cell anemia and thalassemia

Case Scenario

A 5.5-year-old girl presented with cough, dyspnea, irritability, and fatigue. She was underbuilt, under nourished with a short stature, with evident icterus, and yellow tinged fingernails. Child has history of few blood transfusions in the past.

Careful examination revealed maxillary expansion, retracted upper lip and saddle nose and decaying of few upper teeth.

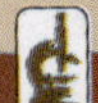

Laboratory Findings Reveal

- Hemoglobin—4.5 g/dL (12–16 g/dL)
- Peripheral blood film revealed microcytic hypochromic anemia with anisocytosis, poikilocytosis, nucleated red blood cells (RBCs)

QUESTIONS

Q.1. What is the most probable diagnosis and cause of above clinical condition?

Q.2. What is the biochemical basis, etiopathogenesis and inheritance of above clinical condition?

Q.3. How you can confirm your diagnosis?

Q.4. What is the line of management of such patients?

ANSWERS

A.1. Child is suffering from thalassemia. Clinical presentation of thalassemia is summarized in **Figure 7.7.1**.

Hemoglobin is made up of heme and globin (protein chains). In adult hemoglobin out of four globin chains two are alpha and two are beta chains **(Flowchart 7.7.1)**.

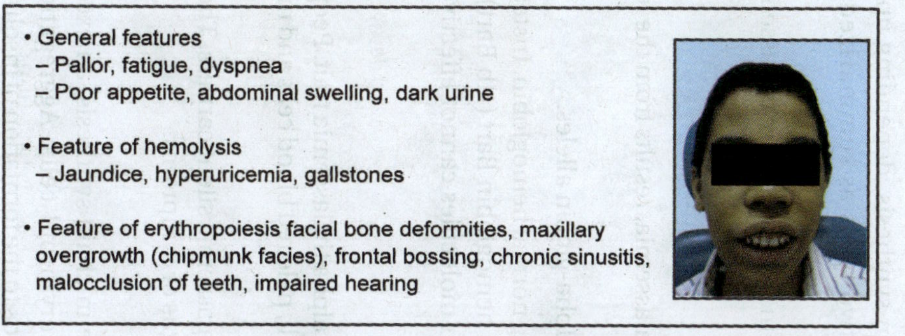

Fig. 7.7.1: Clinical presentation of thalassemia.

Flowchart 7.7.1: Classification of thalassemia.

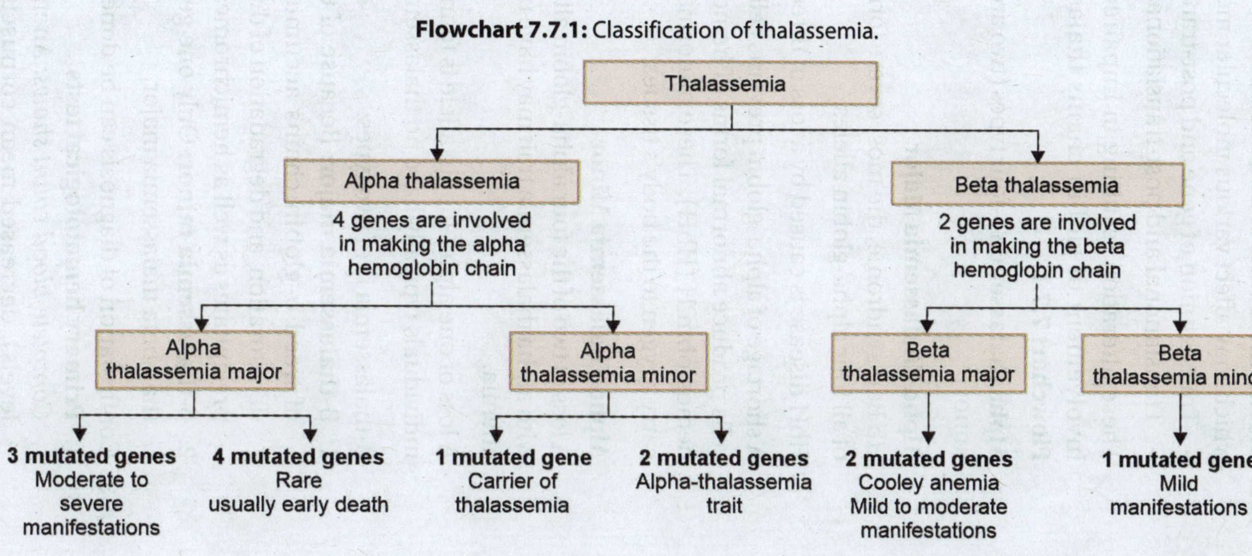

Thalassemia is inherited autosomal recessive disorders characterized by reduced rate of hemoglobin synthesis due to a defect in alpha (α) or beta (β) globin chain synthesis resulting in microcytic hypochromic anemia.

A.2. Biochemical basis of thalassemia: Thalassemia is caused by a spectrum of mutations which may affect various molecular mechanisms which can be:

- Transcription of gene and post-transcriptional modification of mRNA
- Translational and post-translational modification

These alteration resulting in impaired globin chain synthesis, depending upon involvement of globin chains thalassemia is of two types as summarized in **Flowchart 7.7.1**.

Alpha thalassemia—four types (two are thalassemia major and two are thalassemia minor)

Alpha Thalassemia Major

Hb Bart syndrome, the most severe form of alpha thalassemia, results from the loss of all four alpha-globin alleles.

HbH disease is caused by a loss of three of the four alpha-globin alleles.

A shortage of alpha-globin prevents cells from making normal hemoglobin. Instead, cells produce abnormal forms of hemoglobin called hemoglobin Bart (Hb Bart) or hemoglobin H (HbH). These abnormal hemoglobin molecules cannot effectively carry oxygen to the body's tissues.

Alpha Thalassemia Minor

A loss of two of the four alpha-globin alleles results in alpha thalassemia trait. People with alpha thalassemia trait may have unusually small, pale red blood cells and mild anemia.

A loss of one alpha-globin allele is found in alpha thalassemia silent carriers. These individuals typically have no thalassemia-related signs or symptoms.

β-thalassemia is of two types:

1. β-**thalassemia major:** Because of the imbalance in chain synthesis, an excess of freed α-globin chains accumulates within erythroid cells. Aggregation, denaturation, and degradation of these chains leads to the formation of insoluble precipitates as well as hemichromes, which damage cell membranes.
2. β-**thalassemia minor:** Only one gene is affected, symptoms will be less severe than beta thalassemia major.

A.3. Confirmation of diagnosis can be done by three stages approach:

1. **Primary hematological tests**

   Complete blood count shows: Anemia (low blood count, reduced hemoglobin levels), decreased mean corpuscular volume (MCV) and mean corpuscular hemoglobin (MCH).

   Peripheral blood smear shows: Hypochromic microcytic red blood cells, reticulocytosis, target cells, inclusion bodies.

2. **Differentiate types of thalassemia:** Hb electrophoresis, high pressure liquid chromatography (HPLC)
3. **Identification of mutation:** Genetic testing, DNA analysis for α and β globin mutations.

A.4. Line of management for thalassemia patients are as follows:

- Thalassemia minor and traits conditions are either asymptomatic or require only supportive treatment.
- Thalassemia major condition standard treatments for thalassemia major are blood transfusions and iron chelation.

Other available options are:

- Folic acid supplements
- Bone marrow and stem cell transplant
- Luspatercept is a recently approved hematopoietic drug for thalassemia

BIBLIOGRAPHY

1. Bajwa H, Basit H. Thalassemia. In: StatPearls [Internet]. Treasure Island (FL): StatPearls Publishing; 2022.
2. Banjade P, Bhandari J. A child lost to follow up carrying beta thalassemia major: A case report. JNMA J Nepal Med Assoc. 2020;58(226):436-8.

GIVE REASONS WHY

Q.1. Binding of oxygen to heme is a cooperative binding.

Ans. Hemoglobin is usually present in two conformation T (taut form) where all four polypeptide chains of hemoglobin hold together with noncovalent bonds, second is (relaxed) R form, when the noncovalent bonds breaks between the polypeptide chain.

Once O_2 binds to heme in taut form of (deoxygenated) hemoglobin, then binding of O_2 brings iron atom (Fe^{+2}) into the plane of protoporphyrin ring. This movement of Fe^{+2} also moves covalently bind proximal histidine residue of β-globin chain and the movement is transmitted to the proximal polypeptide chains, causes breaking of noncovalent bonds between polypeptide chains. So binding of one O_2 to heme facilitates the binding of next O_2 then further facilitates the binding of 3rd and then 4th O_2 known as positive co-operativity.

Q.2. 2,3 BPG level in RBC increases in high altitude.

Ans. 1,3 BPG is one of the intermediate compound of glycolysis. In RBCs 1,3 BPG is isomerized to 2,3 BPG. This 2,3 BPG decreases O_2 affinity of hemoglobin and favors unloading of O_2 from oxyhemoglobin. That is the reason 2,3 BPG concentration increases in hypoxia, severe anemia and at high attitude.

Q.3. The shape of oxygen dissociation curve (ODC) is sigmoid for hemoglobin, while it is rectangular for myoglobin.

Ans. Oxygen dissociation curve for hemoglobin

Sigmoid nature of graph of ODC for hemoglobin indicates its fractional binding with O_2 at different partial pressure of O_2, also shows that the nature of hemoglobin for readily binds and easily release O_2 whenever required:

- In initial phase when Hb is present in taut form (deoxygenated form) at low O_2 pressure, it is difficult for O_2 to bind with Hb.

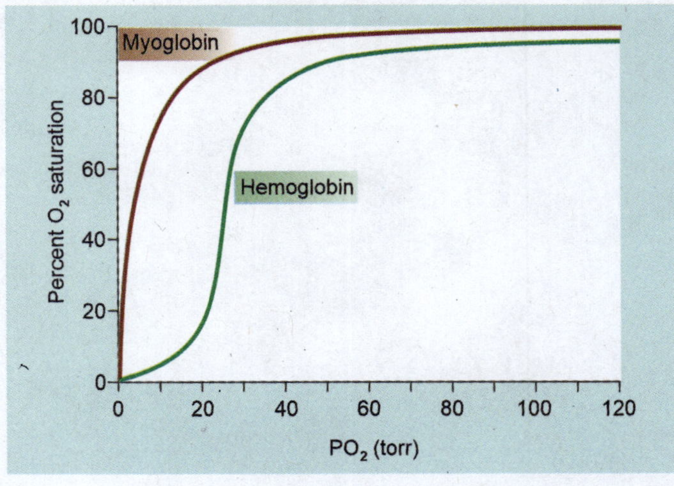

- However, once a molecule of O_2 binds and there is rise in partial pressure of O_2, attachment of O_2 will be through positive cooperativity. At PO_2 (26 turr), 50% of Hb gets saturated with oxygen.
- This process will continue at PO_2 (40 torr)—Hb is 64% saturated.
- In lung capillaries where PO_2 (90 torr)—Hb is 96% saturated.

Oxygen dissociation curve for myoglobin

The shape of graph will be rectangular hyperbola. As myoglobin contains single polypeptide chain. It tightly binds O_2, it has more affinity for O_2 as compared to hemoglobin. It basically act as storage of O_2 in muscle and releases the O_2 when PO_2 at a very low-level of (5 torr) in severe physical exercise. However it is about 50% saturated with oxygen at PO_2 of 1–2 torr.

- High affinity of myoglobin for O_2 at PO_2-40 torr (in resting muscles)
- 95% saturation at PO_2 = 20 torr (in exercising muscle)
- 30% saturation at PO_2–1–2 torr

Q.4. Color of hematoma changes from blue to green and then yellow.

Ans. Venous blood accumulates in hematoma to give it blue color, then further the heme with the action of heme oxygenase, changes to various blood pigment and according produces different color.

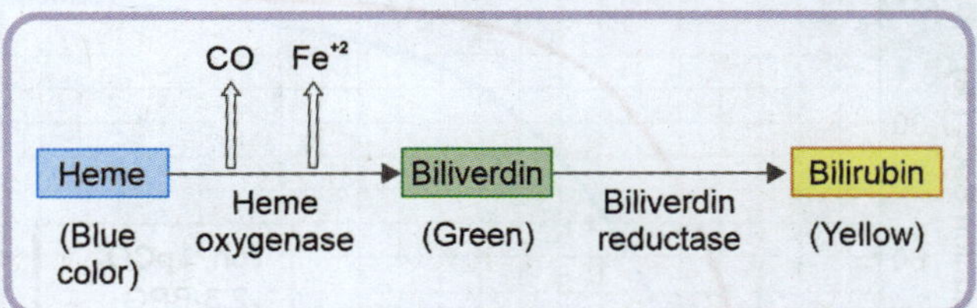

Q.5. Bilirubin does not appear in urine in prehepatic jaundice.

Ans. In prehepatic jaundice unconjugated bilirubin increases in circulation, as it is water insoluble it cannot cross the glomerular filtration membrane and remain absent in urine, however, it's level increases in blood. In circulation in binds with albumin, maximum capacity of albumin to bind is 20 mg/dL after which it can cross the blood brain barrier and gets deposited in the basal ganglia, hippocampus and cerebellum. It is a neurotoxic and causes convulsions, the condition is known as kernicterus. Unconjugated bilirubin is taken up by hepatocytes, where it conjugates with glucuronic acid to form bilirubin monoglucuronide (~10%) bilirubin diglucuronide (~90%), this conjugation makes it water soluble. Conjugate bilirubin though water soluble, it does not regurgitate in circulation until there is obstruction in bile duct. It usually excretes through bile duct in intestine.

Q.6. Certain drugs like barbiturates and phenytoin increase the heme synthesis.

Ans. These drugs are catabolized in the body through cytochrome P450 which is a heme containing enzyme complex, so as heme is used for CYP450 synthesis, its requirement increases in metabolism of various drugs. There will be decrease in co-repression of heme on ALA synthase and enhances its synthesis.

Q.7. Cutaneous manifestation or skin sensitivity is seen in various porphyria.

Ans. In the metabolic pathway of heme synthesis, if defect is below the PBG deaminase porphobilinogen deaminase or uroporphyrinogen I, then any defect in enzymes leads to accumulation of porphobilinogen which further get oxidized to synthesized porphyrins. These porphyrins excreted in urine, gives it pink color or may deposit in teeth (erythrodontia). On exposure with UV rays (near 400 nm), these porphyrins get excited and further form oxygen free radicals. Both of these product damage lysosomes and cause release of lysosomal enzymes results in skin damage, itching, and burning.

Q.8. Fetal hemoglobin (HbF) shows higher oxygen affinity.

Ans. There is a structural difference in HbF and HbA in β-globin chain, at 143 position histidine residue in HbA is replaced with serine in HbF. HbF exhibits a higher affinity for oxygen and a decreased affinity for 2,3-biphosphoglycerate (2,3-BPG). This results in a left-shifted oxyhemoglobin dissociation curve (ODC) of HbF relative to HbA. The leftward shift in the ODC ensures an oxygen uptake at a lower partial oxygen pressure (pO_2) for fetus in utero.

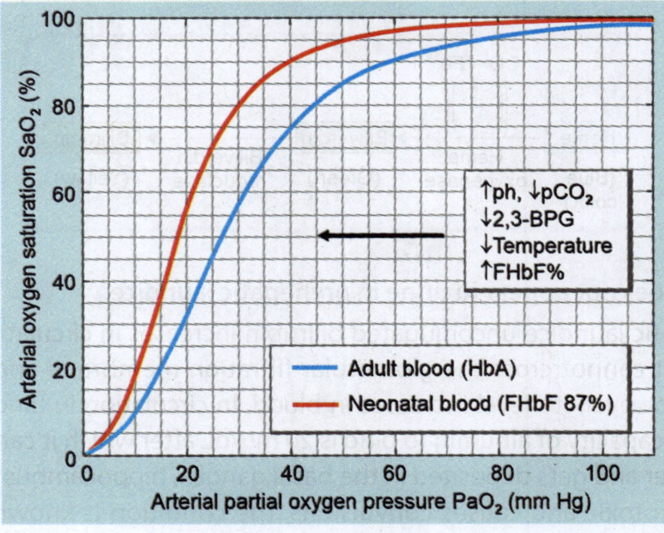

Section 8

Hormones

- **Case 8.1:** Hypothyroidism
- **Case 8.2:** Hyperthyroidism
- **Case 8.3:** Infertility

Give Reasons Why

Case 8.1

Hypothyroidism

COMPETENCY

- ❖ **BC11.1:** Describe the function tests of kidney, liver, thyroid and adrenal glands and their clinical significance. Interpret the function tests report
- ❖ **BC14.19:** Explain the basis and rationale of biochemical tests done and interpretation of laboratory results in Thyroid disorders

Integration with Medicine

- ❖ **GM12.1:** Describe the epidemiology, genetic basis and pathogenesis of hypothyroidism and hyperthyroidism including the influence of iodine deficiency and autoimmunity in the pathogenesis of thyroid disease

Case Scenario

A 50-year-old housewife complains of fatigue, slight memory loss, and constipation, weight gain for last one year. The patient has had diabetes for 15 years being treated with an oral hypoglycemic agent. She is moderately obese and speaks slowly and has a puffy face with pale, cool skin.

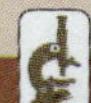

Laboratory Findings Reveal

- Blood glucose—146 mg/dL (70–110 mg/dL)
- Serum total protein—6.8 g/dL, Serum albumin 4.2 g/dL (3.5–5.5 g/dL)
- Serum T3 concentration—0.08 µg/dL (2.3–4.2 pg/mL)
- Serum T4 concentration—1.8 µg/dL (0.8–1.7 ng/dL)
- Serum TSH—10 IU/mL (0.34–4.25 IU/mL)
- Serum cholesterol—255 mg/dL (up to 200 mg/dL)
- Serum urea—48 mg/dL (10–40 mg/dL)
- Serum creatinine—0.8 mg/dL (0.4–1.2 mg/dL)
- CBC and differential WBC are normal

QUESTIONS

Q.1. What is the most probable diagnosis and what are the causes of above clinical condition?

Q.2. What additional aspects of the history and physical examination should be done to exclude differential diagnosis?

Q.3. What are the other investigations required in such a clinical case?

Q.4. What is the line of management of such patients?

ANSWERS

A.1. Patient most probably suffering from hypothyroidism Clinical presentation of hypothyroidism is summarized in **Table 8.1.1**. It is a clinical condition in which the thyroid gland does not produce enough thyroid hormone as per body requirement, it can be classified into:

- Primary hypothyroidism—due to thyroid hormone deficiency
- Secondary hypothyroidism—due to TSH deficiency from pituitary gland
- Tertiary—due to thyrotropin-releasing hormone deficiency
- Peripheral hypothyroidism—thyroid hormone deficiency due to extrathyroidal causes
- Central hypothyroidism—pituitary and hypothalamic disorders

Table 8.1.1: Clinical presentation of hypothyroidism.

Signs	*Symptoms*
• Hypothermia • Bradycardia • Delayed relaxation of deep tendon reflexes • Periorbital edema • Enlargement of tongue • Diastolic hypertension • Hair loss • Pleural and pericardial effusions	• Fatigue • Weakness • Weight gain • Constipation • Cold intolerance • Dry skin • Hoarse voice • Edema • Cognitive dysfunction • Depression • Muscle cramps • Paresthesias • Menorrhagia • Dry, gritty-feeling eyes

Causes of Hypothyroidism

- Autoimmune disorders such as Hashimoto's thyroiditis
- Congenital absence of thyroid gland
- Pituitary disorder (secondary)
- Postpartum hypothyroidism
- Iodine deficiency
- Post-surgical treatment of hyperthyroidism

A.2. Before making diagnosis of such patients, complete evaluation of history and thorough clinical examination should be done to exclude various differential diagnosis as well as to find out other co-existing disorders.

Other differential diagnosis of this patient can be:

- Hypoalbuminemia
- Diabetic nephropathy
- Nephrotic syndrome due to some other causes
- Cirrhosis due to hemochromatosis
- Secondary hypothyroidism

As patients is already diabetic, evaluation related to diabetic control as well as development of any diabetic complication should be sort out—poorer the control, more likely there is diabetic nephropathy, diabetic retinopathy, diabetic cardiovascular complications can occur investigation like glycosylated hemoglobin (HbA1c), serum urea, serum creatinine, urinary albumin creatinine ratio should be done.

For nutritional deficiency disorder, malnutrition investigations like serum total protein, serum albumin, vitamin B_{12}, etc., should be done. Evaluation of any other endocrinal disorder (pituitary-hypothalamic mass, adrenal disorder) proper history of medicine and drugs should be evaluated.

A.3. Thyroid conditions are among the most common endocrine disorders. Laboratory tests are integral in the diagnosis and management of most of these conditions. Other than thyroid function tests investigations which can be useful are:

1. Thyroid imaging, such as thyroid ultrasound or radionuclide scans.
2. Thyroid autoantibodies to diagnose autoimmune thyroid diseases, such as Hashimoto's thyroiditis and Graves' disease.
3. Thyroglobulin (Tg) and calcitonin are used as tumor markers in differentiated thyroid carcinoma (DTC) and medullary thyroid carcinoma.

A.4. Levothyroxine, taken on an empty stomach, is the treatment of choice, women of childbearing age with levothyroxine-treated hypothyroidism should be informed to increase their dose by 30%.

BIBLIOGRAPHY

1. Chaker L, Bianco AC, Jonklaas J, Peeters RP. Hypothyroidism. Lancet. 2017;390(10101):1550-62.
2. Soh SB, Aw TC. Laboratory testing in thyroid conditions—pitfalls and clinical utility. Ann Lab Med. 2019;39(1):3-14.

Case 8.2

Hyperthyroidism

COMPETENCY

- ❖ **BC11.1:** Describe the function tests of kidney, liver, thyroid and adrenal glands and their clinical significance. Interpret the function tests report
- ❖ **BC14.19:** Explain the basis and rationale of biochemical tests done and interpretation of laboratory results in Thyroid disorders

Integration with Medicine

- ❖ **GM12.1:** Describe the epidemiology, genetic basis and pathogenesis of hypothyroidism and hyperthyroidism including the influence of iodine deficiency and autoimmunity in the pathogenesis of thyroid disease

Case Scenario

A 35-year-old nurse complained of nervousness, mood swings, weakness, and palpitations with exertion for the past 6 months. Recently, she noticed weight lose excessive sweating and wanted to sleep with fewer blankets than her husband. Menstrual periods had been regular but there was less bleeding. She appeared anxious, with a smooth, warm, and moist skin and she couldn't rise from a deep knee bend without aid.

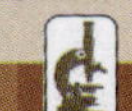

Laboratory Findings Reveal

- Serum T3 = 185 ng/dL (80–220 ng/dL)
- Serum T4 = 15.6 μg/dL
- Serum TSH = 0.001 mIU/L (0.34–4.25 mIU/L)

QUESTIONS

Q.1. What is the most probable diagnosis and cause of above clinical condition?

Q.2. What are the other investigations required to confirm your diagnosis?

Q.3. What is the line of management of such patients?

ANSWERS

A.1. Patient is most probably suffering from hyperthyroidism. Hyperthyroidism defines as condition that occurs when the thyroid gland makes more thyroid hormones than the body needs. Clinical presentation of hyperthyroidism is summarized in **Table 8.2.1**.

Causes of Hyperthyroidism

- Graves' disease, an autoimmune disorder
- Thyroid nodules
- Thyroiditis, inflammation of the thyroid
- Excessive iodine intake
- Drugs like amiodarone

Table 8.2.1: Clinical presentation of hyperthyroidism.

General	**Dermatologic**
• Weight loss	• Pruritus
• Heat intolerance	• Warm/moist skin
• Thyroid enlargement	• Alopecia
• Increased gastrointestinal motility	• Sweating
• Weakness	• Separation of nail from nail bed
• Insomnia	**Central nervous system**
Cardiorespiratory	• Anxiety
• Tachycardia	• Agitation
• Atrial fibrillation	• Restlessness
• Shortness of breath	• Shortness of breath
• Systolic murmur	• Emotional lability
Ocular	• Memory loss
• Burning	• Hyperreflexia
• Irritation	**Reproductive**
• Proptosis	• Oligomenorrhea
• Decreased	• Amenorrhea
• Lid lag	• Gynecomastia
	• Decreased libido

A.2. Confirmation of hyperthyroidism done by thyroid function test including:

- Thyroid function test (T3, T4, TSH, Free T3 and Free T4)
- Additional investigations are imaging tests including radioactive iodine uptake (RAIU) test, thyroid scan, thyroid ultrasound

A.3. Treatment of hyperthyroidism is principally based on:

- Anti-thyroid drugs—methimazole, propylthiouracil
- Radioactive iodine
- Surgery—thyroidectomy
- Beta blockers

BIBLIOGRAPHY

1. de Leo S, Lee SY, Braverman LE. Hyperthyroidism. Lancet. 2016;388(10047):906-18.
2. Kravets I. Hyperthyroidism: Diagnosis and Treatment. Am Fam Physician. 2016;93(5):363-70.

Case 8.3

Infertility

COMPETENCY

- **BC8.5:** Describe the causes (including dietary habits), effects and health risks associated with being overweight/obese/metabolic syndrome
- **BC11.2:** Enumerate the hormones and markers related to reproduction and reproductive health and their clinical interpretation (e.g., LH, FSH, prolactin, beta-HCG, estrogen progesterone, testosterone and AMH). Discuss importance of prenatal screening

Case Scenario

A 37-year-old overweight female and her 37-year-old husband present with the complaint of a possible fertility problem. The couple has been married for 3 years. The patient used birth control pills until one-and-a-half-year-ago. The couple has been trying to conceive since then and report a high degree of stress related to their lack of success. The patient reports good health with normal menstrual history. Past history is remarkable only for mild depression. Imipramine 150 mg three time a day for the last 8 months is her only medication. She works as a cashier and has no history of STDs, abnormal Pap, smoking, alcohol or other drugs. She has had no surgery.

The patient's partner also reports good health and reports no problems. He has had no prior urogenital infections or exposure to STDs. He occasionally uses amphetamines to stay awake while driving at night.

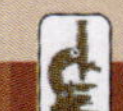

Laboratory Findings Reveal

- T3,T4, TSH normal
- FSH, LH normal
- Prolactin—60 ng/mL (normal range <20 ng/mL)
- Semen analysis of male partner shows normal count and motility of sperm

QUESTIONS

Q.1. What is the definition of infertility?

Q.2. What are the risk factors and causes of infertility?

Q.3. What are the other investigations required to confirm your diagnosis?

ANSWERS

A.1. Couple is defined infertile when they are trying for more than one year (or longer) and female partner not being able to conceive. The contribution of male and female factors is about 40% each. For women, ovulatory failure is the commonest cause (25%), followed by tubal blockage (20%). For men, the commonest cause is sperm defects or dysfunction (30–40%). Unexplained infertility may be as high as 25%.

Types of infertility include:

- **Primary:** A woman who was never pregnant and who cannot conceive after 1 year of not using birth control.
- **Secondary:** Secondary infertility occurs when a woman cannot get pregnant again after having at least one successful pregnancy.

A.2. Factors which can increase the risk of infertility in all both genders are as follows:

- Age (>35 for women or over 40 for men).
- Diabetes.
- Eating disorders, including anorexia nervosa and bulimia nervosa.
- Excessive alcohol use.
- Exposure to environmental toxins, such as lead and pesticides.
- Over-exercising.
- Radiation therapy or other cancer treatments.
- Sexually transmitted diseases (STDs).
- Smoking.
- Stress.
- Substance abuse.
- Weight problems (obesity or underweight).

Causes of infertility: There are various causes of infertility in both genders, these are summarized in **Figures 8.3.1 and 8.3.2.**

Male infertility

Pre-testicular or endocrine causes:
- Unhealthy lifestyle habits
- Diabetes
- Hypothyroidism and hyperthyroidism
- Hypogonadism
- Hyperprolactinemia

Testicular causes:
- **Congenital anomalies or abnormalities:** Genetic alteration is the chromosomal level (i.e., the Klinefelter syndrome)
- **Acquired disorders**: Varicocele, cryptorchidism, orchitiis and hydrocele.

Post-testicular causes: Infections, trauma, anti-sperm antibodies, hypospadias or cystic fibrosis.

Sperm abnormalities: Alterations in the sperm morphology, motility, vitality, or number.
- Oligospermia or oligozoospermia—low sperm count.
- Asthenozoospermia—poor sperm motility.
- Teratospermia or teratozoospermia—large amount of sperm with an abnormal morphology.
- Necrospermia or necrozoospermia—large amount of dead sperm in the ejaculate.
- Azospermia—zero sperm count.

Medicines and drugs: Anabolic hormones, herbal medicines, chemotherapy.

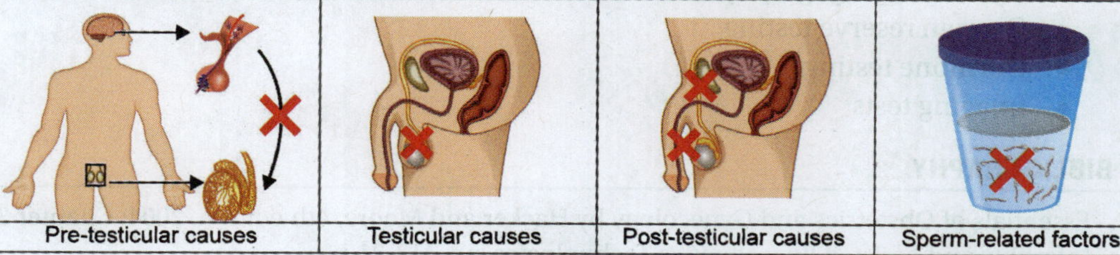

Fig. 8.3.1: Causes of male infertility.

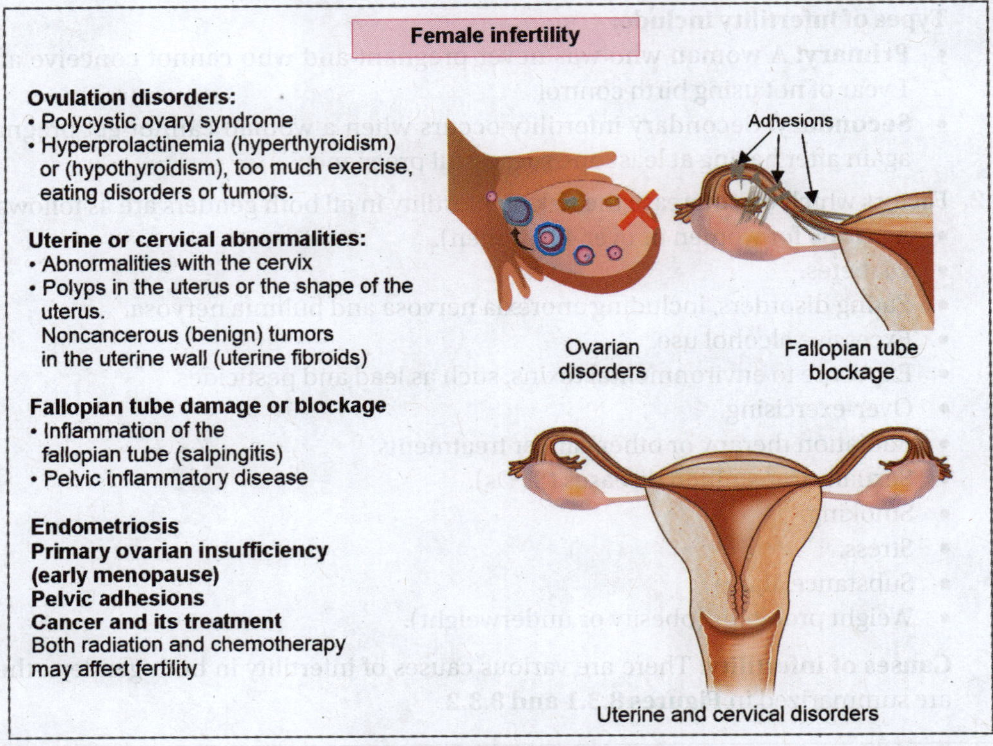

Fig. 8.3.2: Causes of female infertility.

A.3. To find out exact explanations for infertility in either sex, precise investigation approach are available to analysis the root cause of infertility.

Tests for Men

- Semen analysis
- Hormone testing
- Genetic testing
- Testicular biopsy
- Imaging techniques

Tests for Women

- Ovulation testing
- Hysterosalpingography
- Ovarian reserve testing
- Hormone testing
- Imaging tests

BIBLIOGRAPHY

1. Essentials of Obstetrics and Gynecology by Hacker and Moore, 4th edition. 2004; Chapter 35 Infertility and Assisted Reproductive Technologies, pp. 413-21.
2. https://my.clevelandclinic.org/health/diseases.
3. Obstetrics and Gynecology by Beckmann, 5th edition. 2006; Chapter 39 Infertility, pp. 384-95.

GIVE REASONS WHY

Q.1. Deficiency of ADH causes diabetes insipidus.

Ans. Antidiuretic hormone (ADH) is secreted from hypothalamus. It is nonapeptide and also known as vasopressin. It acts on distal tubules of renal nephron. It acts by releasing second messenger C-AMP, which further causes phosphorylation of microtubules and microfilaments. The net effect is reabsorption of water through aquaporins. Deficiency of ADH causes loss of excess water through urine known as diabetes insipidus.

Q.2. Deficiency of steroid hydroxylase leads to adrenogenital syndrome.

Ans. Deficiency of various hydroxylases of steroid synthesis causes deficiency of cortisol, which due to feedback mechanism results in excessive release of ACTH, continuous ACTH secretion causes, adrenal hyperplasia, e.g., deficiency of 25 hydroxylase, complete deficiency of cortisol, results in excess feedback secretion of ACTH, which further results in increase androgen synthesis. This may causes virilization of female child and precocious puberty in male child.

11- hydroxylase deficiency is more fatal and child usually not survive.

Q.3. Tamoxifen is given in treatment of breast cancer.

Ans. As breast cancer is estrogen dependent. Tamoxifen as estrogen receptor antagonist is used to block the estrogen receptor and reduces the proliferation of cancer cells. Same as prostate cancer are androgen dependent. Androgen ablation is used for treatment of prostate cancer.

Q.4. Clomiphene citrate is used in treatment for infertility.

Ans. When high estrogen levels are present, they cause feedback inhibition of estrogen receptors in hypothalamus. Clomiphene citrate is a competitive inhibitor of estrogen and removes this feedback inhibition. It results in increased level of G_nRH, which further consequently enhances FSH and LH level. These two hormones are needed for follicular stimulation and ovulation respectively.

Q.5. β-hCG can be detected in urine 4–5 days after missed menstruation in female of reproductive age.

Ans. Luteinizing hormone (LH) peaks 16 hours before ovulation. This LH surge results in ovulation. After ovulation, corpus luteum then secretes progesterone which maintains the secretary phase of endometrium and prepares the endometrium for implantation of fertilized ovum. If implantation occurs, then the function to maintain progesterone level is shifted from LH to β-hCG. This is why β-hCG level increases in blood, it comes in urine and can be detected 4–5 days after a missed period.

Q.6. Hyperthyroidism seen in Grave's disease.

Ans. Thyroid stimulating immunoglobulins or also known as long action thyroid stimulator found in Grave's disease. These autoantibodies bind to TSH receptor and stimulates these receptors, which are not under feedback control, causes excessive formation and release of TSH, which further causes stimulation of thyroid gland to release of T_3 and T_4.

Q.7. Hypothyroidism seen in Hashimoto's thyroiditis.

Ans. Antibodies are present against thyroglobulin (thyroid hormone binding protein) as well as number of antibodies against follicular cell organelle like antimicrosomal and antinuclear antibodies, which causes destruction of follicular cells and leads to hypothyroidism.

Q.8. Catecholamines are hormones of fight or flight responses.

Ans. **Catecholamines**—epinephrine and norepinephrine these neurotransmitters are synthesized from tyrosine in renal medulla, increase in emergency situations like angers, shock and emotional outburst. Their elevation in blood results in increase in heart rate, blood pressure vasoconstriction and bronchodilation.

Section 9

Water, Electrolyte, and Acid Base Balance

- **Case 9.1:** Dehydration
- **Case 9.2:** Respiratory Acidosis
- **Case 9.3:** Respiratory Alkalosis
- **Case 9.4:** Metabolic Acidosis
- **Case 9.5:** Metabolic Alkalosis

Give Reasons Why

Case 9.1

Dehydration

COMPETENCY

- ❖ **BC9.3:** Describe the processes involved in maintenance of normal pH, water and electrolyte balance of body fluids and the derangements associated with them

Integration with Medicine

- ❖ **GM16.2:** Describe and discuss the acute systemic consequences of diarrhea including its impact on fluid balance

Case Scenario

A previously healthy 5-year-old white boy presents to the emergency department with a 5-day history of nausea, anorexia, weakness, abdominal pain, intermittent diarrhea, and episodes of vomiting. He has no history of fever, respiratory or urinary symptoms, or use of laxatives or diuretics.

On physical examination, child was irritable and listless with sunken eyes and slightly dry mucous membranes.

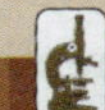

Laboratory Findings Reveal

- Serum sodium—150 mmol/L (136–145 mmol/L)
- Serum urea—70 mg/dL (10–40 mg/dL)
- Serum osmolality—300 mOsm/kg (275–295 mOsm/kg)

QUESTIONS

Q.1. What is the most probable diagnosis and cause of above clinical condition?

Q.2. What are the other investigations useful to confirm your diagnosis?

Q.3. What is the line of management of such patients?

ANSWERS

A.1. Child most probably suffering from dehydration. Clinical presentation of dehydration is summarized in **Figure 9.1.1**.

Other causes of fluid loss (dehydration):

- Blood loss (hemorrhage)
- Excessive vomiting or diarrhea

- Nasogastric suction
- Polyuria (diabetes mellitus, diabetes insipidus)
- Excessive use of laxative or diuretics
- Fever
- Excessive perspiration
- Fluid loss with hemodialysis or peritoneal dialysis

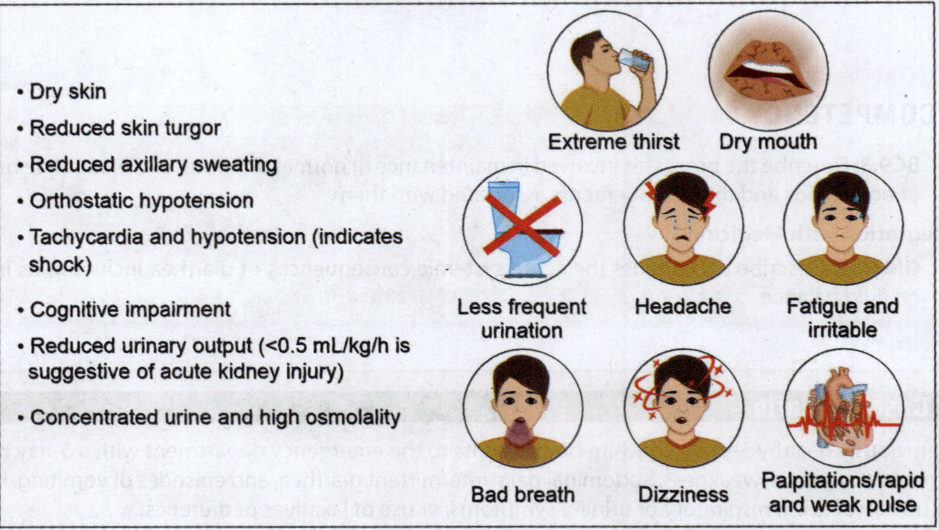

Fig. 9.1.1: Clinical presentation of dehydration.

A.2. Laboratory investigations useful for making diagnosis of dehydration (biochemical changes):
- Raised serum urea
- Raised creatinine
- Reduced or normal estimated glomerular filtration rate (eGFR)
- Hypernatremia (loss of water more than salt loss)
- Raised serum or urine osmolality
- Raised urine specific gravity

A.3. Management of dehydration is depending on grade of dehydration (mild/moderate/severe).

The aim of treatment is to correct the volume and electrolyte deficit as well as keep watch and replace ongoing losses.

BIBLIOGRAPHY

1. Strachan SR, Morris LF. Management of severe dehydration. J Intensive Care Soc. 2017;18(3):251-5.

Case 9.2

Respiratory Acidosis

COMPETENCY

- ❖ **BC9.3:** Describe the processes involved in maintenance of normal pH, water and electrolyte balance of body fluids and the derangements associated with them
- ❖ **BC14.2:** Describe estimation of pH-by-pH meter or ABG analyser and interpretation of results with paper case scenarios

Integration with Medicine

- ❖ **GM23.10:** Enumerate the causes and describe the clinical and laboratory features of respiratory acidosis

Case Scenario

A 68-year-old man with a history of very severe chronic obstructive pulmonary disease (COPD) presents to the emergency room complaining of worsening dyspnea and an increase in the frequency and purulence of his sputum production over the past 2 days. His oxygen saturation is 78% of the room air. Before he is placed on supplemental oxygen, a sample for arterial blood gas analysis is drawn.

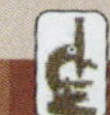

Laboratory Findings Reveal

- pH 7.20 (7.35–7.45)
- PCO_2 68 (40–45 mm of Hg)
- PO_2 48 (80–100 mm of Hg)
- HCO_3^- 31 (22–26 mmol/L)

QUESTIONS

Q.1. What is the most probable diagnosis and cause of above clinical condition?

Q.2. What is the biochemical basis of above clinical condition?

Q.3. What is the line of management of such patients?

ANSWERS

A.1. Patient is suffering from respiratory acidosis. The patient has a low pH (acidemia). The patient has high PCO_2 (respiratory acidosis) and a high bicarbonate (metabolic alkalosis). More precisely patient suffering from respiratory acidosis with compensatory metabolic alkalosis. Clinical presentation of respiratory acidosis is summarized in **Table 9.2.1**.

Causes of Respiratory Acidosis

- **Central respiratory depression:** Stroke, sedative drugs misuse, alcohol overuse
- **Airway obstruction:** Obstructed airways (due to choking or other causes), foreign body, sleep apnea, aspiration, bronchospasm

Table 9.2.1: Clinical presentation of respiratory acidosis.

More common	*Less common*
• Confusion • Anxiety • Being easily fatigued • Lethargy • Memory loss • Shortness of breath • Tremors (shaking or jerking muscle movements) • Warm and flushed skin • Sweating	• Headaches • Altered mental state • Heart failure • Pulmonary hypertension (high blood pressure) • Seizures • Coma

- **Respiratory disorders:** Chronic airway problems or long-term lung disorders such as asthma, chronic obstructive pulmonary disease (COPD), emphysema or pneumonia, pulmonary edema, fibrosis
- Neuromuscular conditions such as myasthenia gravis, muscular dystrophy, or multiple sclerosis
- Conditions that influence the muscles involved in breathing, such as Guillain-Barre syndrome or muscular dystrophy
- Chest injury, deformed chest structure (such as kyphosis), scoliosis or muscle weakness in the chest
- Obesity
- Cardiac arrest

A.2. Biochemical basis of respiratory acidosis.
CO_2 gas is acidic is nature, due to any reason, if CO_2 get accumulated (PCO_2 increased) in blood it will cause dropping of pH which result in respiratory acidosis.

A.3. The primary aim of management if patients is to gradually correct the hypercapnia (high CO_2 in blood). The hypercapnia should be corrected gradually because rapid alkalization of the cerebrospinal fluid (CSF) may lead to seizures. Patients who are lethargic, or confused need to be monitored in the intensive care unit (ICU). Those who exhibit hypoventilation will need endotracheal intubation and mechanical ventilation.

Pharmacologic therapy can also be used to help improve ventilation. Bronchodilators like beta-agonists, anticholinergic drugs, and methylxanthines can be used in treating patients with obstructive airway diseases. Naloxone can be used in patients who overdose on opioid use.

BIBLIOGRAPHY

1. Epstein SK, Singh N. Respiratory acidosis. Respir Care. 2001;46(4):366-83.
2. Patel S, Sharma S. Respiratory Acidosis. [Updated 2022 Jun 21]. In: StatPearls [Internet]. Treasure Island (FL): StatPearls Publishing; 2022. Available from: https://www.ncbi.nlm.nih.gov/books/NBK482430.

Case 9.3

Respiratory Alkalosis

COMPETENCY

- ❖ **BC9.3:** Describe the processes involved in maintenance of normal pH, water and electrolyte balance of body fluids and the derangements associated with them
- ❖ **BC14.2:** Describe estimation of pH-by-pH meter or ABG analyser and interpretation of results with paper case scenarios

Integration with Medicine

- ❖ **GM23.11:** Enumerate the causes and describe the clinical and laboratory features of respiratory alkalosis

Case Scenario

A 52-year-old man comes to the emergency department complaining of shortness of breath and tingling in fingers. He is retired and living alone, his breathing is shallow and rapid. There is no any history of diabetes, hypertension and any other systemic illness. History reveals that he was on several antianxiety medications and also had anxiety attacks before. While being worked up for chest pain, an ABG is done.

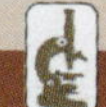

Laboratory Findings Reveal

- pH = 7.48 (7.35–7.45)
- $PaCO_2$ = 28 (40–45 mm of Hg)
- HCO_3 = 22 (22–26 mmol/L)
- PaO_2 = 85 (80–100 mm of Hg)
- PO_2 = 90 mm of Hg (80–100 mm of Hg)

QUESTIONS

Q.1. What is the most probable diagnosis and cause of above clinical condition?

Q.2. What can be the other clinical diagnosis (differential diagnosis) for this clinical presentation?

Q.3. What is the line of management of such patients?

ANSWERS

A.1. Patients is suffering from respiratory alkalosis, respiratory alkalosis is a clinical condition that is secondary to hyperventilation. Clinical presentation of respiratory alkalosis is summarized in **Table 9.3.1**.

Table 9.3.1: Clinical presentation of respiratory alkalosis.

• Paresthesia • Circumoral numbness • Chest pain or tightness • Dyspnea • Confusion • Muscle cramps	• Arrhythmias • Hypokalemia • Hypophosphatemia • Hypocalcemia • Seizures • Tetany

Causes of respiratory alkalosis are:

- Anxiety or pain
- Sepsis
- Central nervous system stimulation (amphetamine overdose)
- Aspirin overdose
- Pregnancy
- Cirrhosis
- Hypoxemia
- Hyperthyroidism

A.2. There are few other clinical conditions which can mimic or result in same clinical presentation, so other possibilities include:

- Asthma exacerbation
- Atrial fibrillation
- Atrial flutter
- Atrial tachycardia
- Bacterial pneumonia
- Bacterial sepsis
- Community-acquired pneumonia
- COPD exacerbation
- Head trauma
- Heatstroke
- Hyperthyroidism and thyrotoxicosis
- Idiopathic pulmonary fibrosis
- Meningitis
- Metabolic alkalosis
- Myocardial infarction
- Panic disorder
- Pneumothorax
- Pulmonary edema/embolism
- Salicylate toxicity
- Theophylline toxicity
- Viral pneumonia

A.3. Respiratory alkalosis itself is not life-threatening and management is based on the underlying etiology, other supportive treatments may include:

- Administering an opioid pain reliever or anti-anxiety medication to reduce hyperventilation

- Providing oxygen to help keep a person from hyperventilating
- Correcting any heart rhythm abnormalities by using medications.

BIBLIOGRAPHY

1. Brinkman JE, Sharma S. Respiratory alkalosis. [Updated 2022 Jul 25]. In: StatPearls [Internet]. Treasure Island (FL): StatPearls Publishing; 2022. Available from: https://www.ncbi.nlm.nih.gov/books/NBK482117/
2. Foster GT, Vaziri ND, Sassoon CS. Respiratory alkalosis. Respir Care. 2001;46(4):384-91.
3. https://www.medicalnewstoday.com/

Case 9.4

Metabolic Acidosis

COMPETENCY

- **BC9.3:** Describe the processes involved in maintenance of normal pH, water and electrolyte balance of body fluids and the derangements associated with them
- **BC14.2:** Describe estimation of pH-by-pH meter or ABG analyser and interpretation of results with paper case scenarios

Integration with Medicine

- **GM23.8:** Enumerate the causes and describe the clinical and laboratory features of metabolic acidosis

Case Scenario

The patient is a 35-year-old female with AIDS brought to the emergency room with a fever of 39°C and three months history of copious diarrhea. On examination, she was in moderate distress with a respiratory rate of 18/minute. There were no any sign of cyanosis, clubbing, or edema. Neurological examination was normal.

Laboratory Findings Reveal

		Normal Values	Arterial Blood Gas
Sodium	136	136–145 mmol/L	pH: 7.2 PCO_2: 30 mmHg PO_2: 90 mmHg Bicarbonate: 14 mmol/L
Potassium	3.4	3.5–5 mmol/L	
Chloride	112	96–106 mmol/L	
Total CO_2	14	23–27 mmol/L	
BUN	30	7–22 mg/dL	
Creatinine	1.5	0.4–1.2 mg/dL	
Glucose	105	70–110 mg/dL	

QUESTIONS

Q.1. What is the most probable diagnosis and cause of above clinical condition?

Q.2. How could you reach on your diagnosis in such clinical condition?

Q.3. What is the line of management of such patients?

ANSWERS

A.1. Patients is most probably suffering from metabolic acidosis. More precisely metabolic acidosis with compensatory respiratory alkalosis. Clinical presentation of metabolic acidosis is summarized in **Table 9.4.1**.

Table 9.4.1: Clinical presentation of metabolic acidosis.	
Breath faster and deeper	Headache
Confusion	Anorexia
Fast heartbeat	Feeling tired
Feeling sick	

Metabolic acidosis is characterized by an increase in the hydrogen ion concentration in the systemic circulation resulting in a serum HCO_3 less than 24 mEq/L. Metabolic acidosis is not a benign condition and signifies an underlying disorder that needs to be corrected to minimize morbidity and mortality.

Cause of Metabolic Acidosis

Metabolic acidosis can be classified into high anion gap acidosis and normal anion gap acidosis as given in **Table 9.4.2**.

Table 9.4.2: Metabolic acidosis classification.

Acidosis	*Metabolic*	
High anion gap acidosis (CAT MUDPILES)	Normal anion gap acidosis	Low anion gap acidosis
C: Cyanide and carbon monoxide poisoning	Gastrointestinal loses of HCO_3 (diarrhea, enteric fistula)	Ingestion of bromide
A: Arsenic	Ureteral diversions (ureterosigmoidostomy, ileal bladder)	Albumin (low)
T: Toluene	Renal tubular acidosis	Multiple myeloma
M: Methanol, metformin	Hyperalimentation	
U: Uremia	Addison's disease	
D: DKA	Medications (acetazolamide, amphotericin-B, ammonium chloride)	
P: Paraldehyde		
I: Iron, INH		
L: Lactate		
E: Ethylene glycol		
S: Salicylates		

A.2. There are certain steps to determine acid-base imbalance, these are summarized as follows:

- Look at the pH
  - It is the primary problem acidosis (low) or alkalosis (high)
- Check the CO_2 (respiratory indicator)
  - It is less than 35 (alkalosis) or more than 45 (acidosis)
- Check the HCO_3 (metabolic indicator)
  - It is less than 22 (acidosis) or more than 26 (alkalosis)
- Which is the primary disorder (respiratory or metabolic)?

- If the pH is low (acidosis), then look to see if CO_2 or HCO_3 is acidosis (whichever is acidosis will be primary).
- If the pH is high (alkalosis), then look to see if CO_2 or HCO_3 is alkalosis (whichever is alkalosis is the primary).

To reach on a conclusion a simple flowchart shown in **Flowchart 9.4.1** will be helpful.

Flowchart 9.4.1: Classification of simple (not mixed) acid-base disorders.

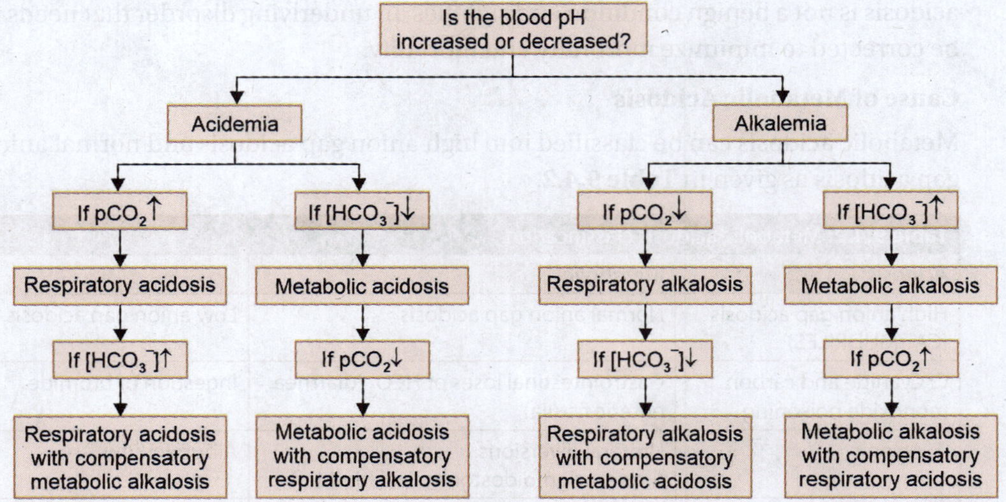

A.3. The management of metabolic acidosis should address the cause of the underlying acid-base derangement. For example, adequate fluid resuscitation and correction of electrolyte abnormalities are necessary for sepsis and diabetic ketoacidosis. Other therapies to consider include antidotes for poisoning, dialysis, antibiotics, and bicarbonate administration in certain situations.

BIBLIOGRAPHY

1. Burger MK, Schaller DJ. Metabolic acidosis. [Updated 2022 Jul 19]. In: StatPearls [Internet]. Treasure Island (FL): StatPearls Publishing; 2022. Available from: https://www.ncbi.nlm.nih.gov/books/NBK482146/
2. Lim S. Metabolic acidosis. Acta Med Indones. 2007;39(3):145-50.

Case 9.5

Metabolic Alkalosis

COMPETENCY

- ❖ **BC9.3:** Describe the processes involved in maintenance of normal pH, water and electrolyte balance of body fluids and the derangements associated with them
- ❖ **BC14.2:** Describe estimation of pH-by-pH meter or ABG analyser and interpretation of results with paper case scenarios

Integration with Medicine

- ❖ **GM23.9:** Enumerate the causes and describe the clinical and laboratory features of metabolic alkalosis

Case Scenario

A 45-year-old man was admitted to the hospital with a history of persistent vomiting. He had a long history of dyspepsia but had never sought advice for this. On examination he was dehydrated with shallow respiration.

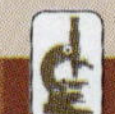

Laboratory Findings Reveal

- pH: 7.56 (7.35–7.45)
- PCO_2: 48 mm Hg (40–45 mm of Hg)
- HCO_3^-: 45 mmol/L (22–26 mmol/L)
- PO_2: 90 mm of Hg (80–100 mm of Hg)

QUESTIONS

Q.1. What is the most probable diagnosis and cause of above clinical condition?

Q.2. What other electrolyte disturbance can co-exist in such clinical condition?

Q.3. What is the line of management of such patients?

ANSWERS

A.1. Patient is suffering from metabolic alkalosis, more precisely metabolic alkalosis with compensatory respiratory acidosis. Clinical presentation of metabolic alkalosis is summarized in **Table 9.5.1**.

Table 9.5.1: Clinical presentation of metabolic alkalosis.	
• Hypoventilation and/or hypoxia • Confusion can progress to coma • Tremor, tingling and numbness • Muscle weakness and twitching	• Prolong muscle spasm (tetany) • Arrhythmias • Nausea, vomiting

Metabolic alkalosis is defined as a disease state where the body's pH is elevated to more than 7.45 and the causes of metabolic alkalosis are given in **Table 9.5.2**.

Table 9.5.2: Causes of metabolic alkalosis.

Gastrointestinal loss of H^+ ions	• Vomiting • Nasogastric suction
Renal loss of H^+ ions	• Mineralocorticoid loss (primary) • Diuretic use (loop and thiazide diuretics) • Hypocalcemia • Milk alkali syndrome • Post-hypercapnic alkalosis
Alkali administration	• Citrate • Cocaine abuse
Hypovolemic (contraction) alkalosis	• Over use of diuretics • Villous adenoma • Factitious diarrhea
Genetic causes	• Bartter's syndrome • Gitelman's syndrome
Electrolyte disturbance	• Hypokalemia

A.2. In metabolic alkalosis severe loss of gastrointestinal fluid due to vomiting result in water depletion (hypervolemia), sodium depletion (hypernatremia), intracellular shifting of potassium (hypokalemia).

Metabolic alkalosis may also be associate with symptoms of hypomagnesemia, hypocalcemia and hypophosphatemia.

A.3. The primary aim in management of metabolic alkalosis is to find out underlying cause of alkalosis and remove it.

Other symptomatic measures are:

- Saline infusion
- Potassium replacement
- Magnesium replacement
- Correct water and electrolyte disturbance
- Stopping the medications that caused the condition, for example high doses of diuretics.

BIBLIOGRAPHY

1. Brinkman JE, Sharma S. Physiology, aetabolic alkalosis. [Updated 2022 Jul 18]. In: StatPearls [Internet]. Treasure Island (FL): StatPearls Publishing; 2022. Available from: https://www.ncbi.nlm.nih.gov/books/NBK482291/
2. Tinawi M. Pathophysiology, evaluation, and management of metabolic alkalosis. Cureus. 2021;13(1):e12841.

GIVE REASONS WHY

Q.1. Water is a good solvent.

Ans. Water is a good solvent because of its dipolar nature. It tends to dissolve common salt as well organic compounds with polar groups (sugar, alcohol, etc.). Water has a tendency to form hydrogen bonds with hydroxyl (-OH), ketone (-C=O), aldehyde (-CHO) group.

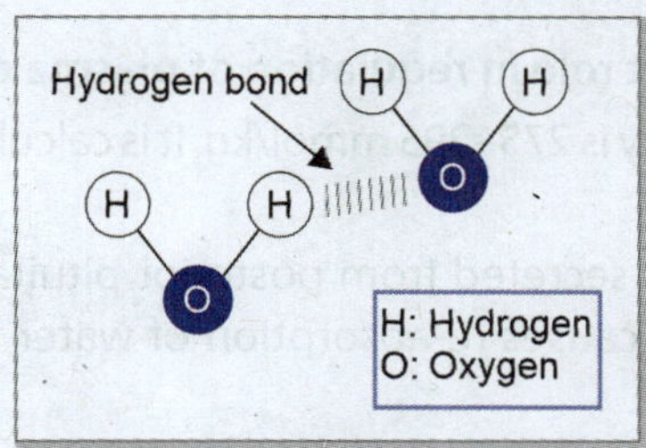

Q.2. Ionic product of water is 1×10^{-14}.

Ans. The equilibrium constant or the dissociation constant of water is expressed as:

- K_{eq} I = ([H^+][OH^-])/H_2O
- The molar concentration of water at equilibrium is 1,000/18 = (Number of grams of water in 1L)/(Gram molecular weight of water) = 55.5
- K_{eq} I by electrical conductivity is 1.8×10^{-16} mol/L (at 25°C)
- $1.8 \times 10^{-16} \times 55.5 = [H^+]\,[OH^-]$
- $1 \times 10^{-14} = [H^+]\,[OH^-]$ = KW (ionic product of water)

Q.3. Why does the salt/acid ratio has to maintain at 20:1 and 4:1 for bicarbonate and phosphate buffer respectively?

Ans. This can be explained by using Henderson-Hasselbalch equation

pH = pKa + Log salt/Acid

As we need to maintain blood pH 7.35-7.45 (average 7.4)

a. For bicarbonate buffer

pH= 6.1+Log 20/1 [HCO_3^-])/H_2CO_3 pKa of $H_2PO_4^{-1}$ = 6.1 = 6.1 + 1.3

b. For phosphate buffer

pH = 6.8 + Log 4/1 [$HPO_4]^{-1}$/[$H_2PO_4]^{-2}$ Pka of [$H_2PO_4]^{-2}$ = 6.8 = 6.8 + 0.6

Q.4. Hyperventilation serves as the major compensatory process in metabolic acidosis, while renal response plays an important role in respiratory acidosis.

Ans. Metabolic acidosis is due to excess formation of organic acids or loss of bicarbonate take place. CO_2 is acidic in nature, so for maintenance the blood pH, CO_2 is exhaled more results in reduction of H_2CO_3 levels/PCO_2 to maintain the ratio of $\frac{HCO_3}{H_2CO_3}$ at $\frac{20}{1}$

In respiratory acidosis, decrease alveolar ventilation results in accumulation of CO_2 and increase in pCO_2 results in acidosis. As lungs cannot compensate the acidosis further compensation can be done only by renal mechanism:

1. Excretion of excess H^+ ions
2. Reabsorption of [HCO_3^-]
3. Excretion of titratable acids
4. Excretion of ammonium ions.

Q.5. ADH plays an important role in regulation of plasma osmolality.

Ans. Normal plasma osmolality is 275–295 mmol/kg. It is calculated as—2 x Na^+ + Glucose/18 + BUN/2.8

Antidiuretic hormone is secreted from posterior pituitary in response to increase in osmolality of plasma. It causes re-absorption of water from renal tubules and bring the osmolality at normal.

Q.6. Renin plays important role in regulation of water and electrolytes.

Ans. Renin hormone secreted from juxtaglomerular cells (JGCs) (a cellular complex) in renal tubules. It is secreted in response to decrease renal blood flow. Further it acts on a protein angiotensinogen secreted from liver and releases a decapeptide angiotensinogen-1 which by action of another peptidase (ACE-angiotensin converting enzyme, secreted from lungs) removes two more amino acids and the remaining octapeptide is known as angiotensin-II. This angiotensin-II causes—vasoconstriction and subsequent rise in blood pressure. It also stimulates synthesis and release of aldosterone from adrenal cortex. Aldosterone causes retention of sodium and water and restore the circulating blood volume.

Section

10 Nucleic Acid Metabolism

- **Case 10.1:** Gout
- **Case 10.2:** Lesch-Nyhan Syndrome
- **Case 10.3:** Nucleoside Analogues as Anticancer Drugs

Give Reasons Why

Case 10.1

Gout

COMPETENCY

- ❖ **BC10.2:** Describe briefly synthesis of purines in the body with special stress on salvage pathway
- ❖ **BC10.3:** Describe the degradation of purines and its significance with associated disorders

Integration with Medicine

- ❖ **GM7.3:** Develop a systematic clinical approach to joint pain based on the pathophysiology

Case Scenario

A 45-year-old male presented to orthopedic OPD with history of pain and swelling in big toe. He consumes alcohol and nonvegetarian. He gave a history of occasional such pain particularly after a night before. On examination, the big toe and ankle looked swollen, red and tender. His blood investigations showed uric acid levels of 8.8 mg/dL.

QUESTIONS

Q.1. What is the suspected diagnosis? Explain the biochemical basis for the clinical symptoms.

Q.2. What is the biochemical basis of clinical presentation of gouty patients, enumerate the risk factors associated with this clinical condition?

Q.3. How alcohol consumption and nonvegetarian diet affect blood uric acid level. What differential diagnosis for this clinical condition?

Q.4. What is the line of management of such clinical condition?

ANSWERS

A.1. Patient is most probably suffering from acute gouty arthritis. Gout is a clinical syndrome characterized by gouty arthritis, gouty nephropathy and subcutaneous accumulation of urate known as "tophi". Clinical presentation of gout is summarized in **Figure 10.1.1**.

Gout is characterized biochemically by extracellular fluid urate saturation, which is reflected by hyperuricemia in the blood, with plasma or serum urate concentrations exceeding 6.8 mg/dL (approximately 400 mmol/L); this level is the approximate limit of urate solubility. The clinical manifestations of gout may include:

- Acute gout flare (recurrent flares of inflammatory arthritis)
- Chronic gouty arthropathy

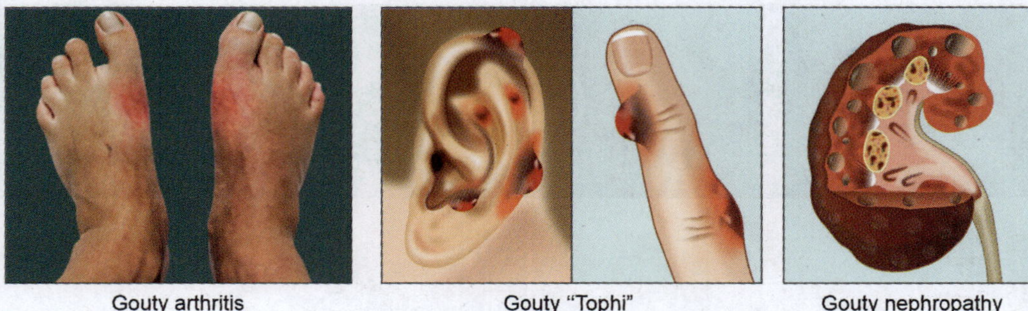

Fig. 10.1.1: Clinical presentation of gout.

- Accumulation of urate crystals in the form of tophaceous deposits
- Uric acid nephrolithiasis
- Chronic nephropathy

This condition most often affecting middle aged to elderly men and postmenopausal women. This condition is usually due to increases in body pool of urate with hyperuricemia. It is typically characterized by deposition of monosodium urate (MSU) crystals in joints and connective tissue (tophi). The first metatarsophalangeal joint of the first toe is usually involved, however other joints like tarsal joints, ankles and knees are also involved. Inflamed Heberden's or Bouchard's nodes may be the first manifestation of gouty arthritis. Episodes of gout usually begins at night with severe pain and swelling of joints.

Types of Gout

Primary—genetic causes having familial inheritance.

- Phosphoribosylpyrophosphate (PRPP) synthetase overactivity
- Glucose-6-phosphatase deficiency
- Deficiency of HGPRTase

Secondary Hyperuricemia (Acquired Reason)

- **Increased production of uric acid:** Malignancy—leukemia, lymphomas, polycythemia (increase breakdown cells leads to the purine degradation and increased uric acid levels).
- Tissue damage due to trauma or as a result of starvation.

Reduced Excretion Rate

- Renal failure
- Diuretics that reduce the secretion of uric acid
- Lactic acidosis/ketoacidosis again interfere with tubular secretion of uric acid.

A.2. Biochemical Basis of Gouty Complications

Uric acid is a weak organic acid. It exists in the ionized form (urate) and nonionized form (uric acid). At pH of 5.5 (pKa of uric acid) half molecules remain in uric acid form and half remain in monosodium urate. At physiological pH 7.4 all the molecules remain in monosodium urate form.

Solubility of these molecules in blood depend upon blood pH and temperature:

1. **Blood pH:** Uric acid is barely soluble in nature, its solubility increases in blood with increase in pH and decrease in acidic pH. In acid fluids like urine, uric acid exists in the nonionized form (uric acid), which is less soluble. This explains the presence of uric acid crystals and stones in the urinary tract in distinction to MSU.
   While as pH increases monosodium urate, which is present in abundance starts getting saturated (solubility of monosodium urate has a minimum near pH 7.7 at 37°C) and deposited in form of monosodium crystal in joints and connective tissue (tophi).
2. **Temperature:** Decreased in temperature decrease solubility of monosodium urate, result in crystallization at cooler body parts (great toe, pinna, subcutaneous tissue).

Risk Factors

Hyperuricemia is not the only risk factor for gout, and in fact, only a minority of these patients develop gout. Dietary sources that can contribute to hyperuricemia and gout include the consumption of animal food such as seafood (e.g., shrimp, lobster), organs (e.g., liver and kidney), and red meat (pork, beef). Some drinks like alcohol, sweetened beverages, sodas, and high-fructose corn syrup may also contribute to these diseases.

Other factors implicated in gout and/or hyperuricemia include older age, male sex, obesity, a purine diet, alcohol, medications, comorbid diseases, and a sedentary lifestyle and genetics. Medications include diuretics, low-dose aspirin, ethambutol, pyrazinamide, and cyclosporine can precipitate the acute attack.

A.3. Excess intake of alcohol lead to production of lactic acid, which causes decrease in blood pH, acidic pH lowers the solubility of uric acid as well as lactic acid competes with uric acid for excretion which cause hyperuricemia. Mechanism of alcohol metabolism is summarized in **Figure 10.1.2**.

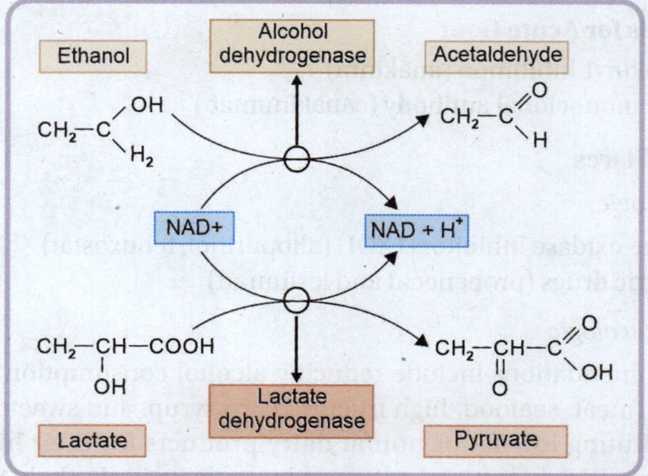

Fig. 10.1.2: Alcohol metabolism.

Nonvegetarian Diet

Consuming animal-based foods that are high in purines increase the risk of developing gout, because the body metabolize purines into uric acid.

Differential Diagnosis of Gout

Gout flare

- Pseudogout (calcium pyrophosphate crystal deposition) disease
- Basic calcium phosphate crystal disease
- Septic arthritis
- Osteoarthritis
- Psoriatic arthritis
- Cellulitis
- Trauma

Tophaceous gout

- Dactylitis
- Rheumatoid arthritis
- Osteomyelitis

A.4. **Managment of gout** is based on clinical status of patients. During acute flares, the goal is solely to reduce the inflammation and symptoms. Long-term goal is to reduce serum urate levels to achieve suppression of flare-ups and regression of gouty complications.

Acute Gout Flare

Management of acute flares aims at decreasing the inflammation and the resulting pain treatment should be started within the first 24 hours of onset to reduce the severity and duration of the flare-up. First-line treatments for gout flares are NSAIDs, (nonsteroidal anti-inflammatory drugs) colchicine, or systemic glucocorticoids.

Prophylaxis for Acute Gout

- Interleukin-1 inhibition (anakinra)
- Specific monoclonal antibody (canakinumab)

Nonacute Flares

Pharmacologic

- Xanthine oxidase inhibitors (XOI) (allopurinol, febuxostat)
- Uricosuric drugs (probenecid and lesinurad)

Nonpharmacologic

Diet recommendations include reducing alcohol consumption, limiting purine-rich foods (meat, seafood, high fructose corn syrup, and sweetened soft drinks), and substituting low-fat or nonfat dairy products for their higher fat content counterparts. Weight loss and adequate hydration will also help reduce gout flare-up frequency.

BIBLIOGRAPHY

1. Fenando A, Rednam M, Gujarathi R, et al. Gout. [Updated 2022 May 21]. In: StatPearls [Internet]. Treasure Island (FL): StatPearls Publishing; 2022 Jan-. Available from: https://www.ncbi.nlm.nih.gov/books/NBK546606/
2. Perez-Ruiz F, Castillo E, Chinchilla SP, Herrero-Beites AM. Clinical manifestations and diagnosis of gout. Rheum Dis Clin North Am. 2014;40(2):193-206.

Case 10.2

Lesch-Nyhan Syndrome

COMPETENCY

- ❖ **BC10.2:** Describe briefly synthesis of purines in the body with special stress on salvage pathway
- ❖ **BC10.3:** Describe the degradation of purines and its significance with associated disorders

Case Scenario

A 2-year-old boy was admitted in pediatric ward, because of severe and repeated lip chewing and aggressive tongue biting, history revealed a normal childbirth with no complications but a diagnosis of muscular hypotonia was made at 5 months of age.

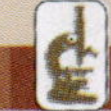

Laboratory Findings Reveal

- Serum uric acid—11 mg/dL (3–7 mg/dL)

QUESTIONS

Q.1. What is the most probable diagnosis of this this case?

Q.2. What are the biochemical basis of clinical presentation in this condition?

Q.3. What is the line of management of such a clinical disorder?

ANSWERS

A.1. Child is suffering with LNS (Lesch-Nyhan syndrome). It is a rare X-linked disorder characterized by dystonia, spasticity, intellectual disability, and self-mutilation. Clinical presentation of Lesch-Nyhan syndrome is summarized in **Figure 10.2.1**.

- Self-mutilating behavior
- Moderate mental retardation
- Spasticity
- Chorea—purpose less repetitive movements
- Athetosis—uncontrolled spastic muscle movements
- Dysphagia, irritability
- Urate crystals looks like orange sand in diaper of children
- Swelling in joint, vomiting

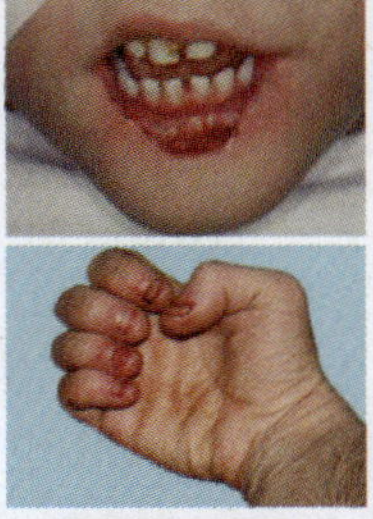

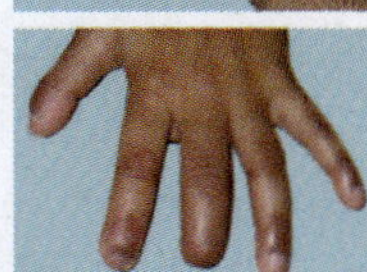

Fig. 10.2.1: Clinical presentation of Lesch-Nyhan syndrome.

A.2. Lesch-Nyhan syndrome is associated with deficiency of HGPRTase (hypoxanthine-guanine phosphoribosyl transferase) one of the enzyme of salvage pathway of purine synthesis. This is X-linked inherited disorder, so occurrence is most common in males (incidence 1:10,000). This pathway is crucial for some tissues, such as RBCs and brain, where de novo synthesis of purine synthesis is not functional. These organs have low activity of PRPP amidotransferase (committed step for de novo synthesis) and are dependent on the salvage pathway for the requirement of nucleotides take IMP and GMP.

Delayed milestone, self-mutilation and bleeding disorder are due to reduced activity of salvage pathway in brain and RBCs.

One hypothesis is the accelerated biosynthesis of semi-essential amino acid histidine that against the background of accelerated purine de novo biosynthesis results in 5-aminoimidazole-4-carboxamide ribonucleotide (AICAR) and histamine accumulation. The histamine and AICAR were determined to be the compounds that cause the neurobehavioral symptoms of LNS **(Fig. 10.2.2)**.

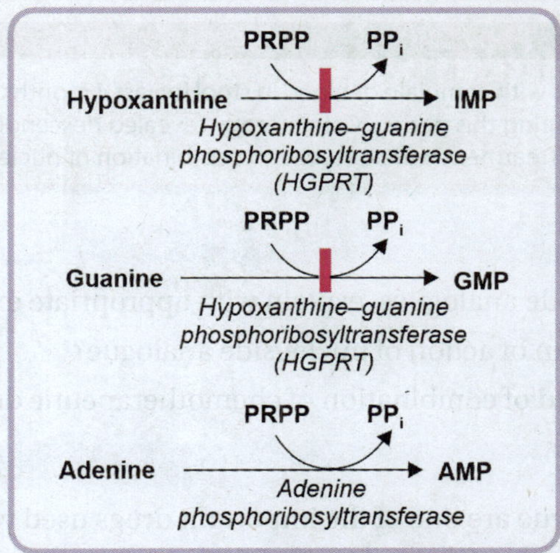

Fig. 10.2.2: Purine metabolic salvage pathway.

A.3. There is no specific treatment for LNS. Xanthine oxidase inhibitors are given to reduce high level of uric acid. Spasticity and dystonia can be managed with benzodiazepines (diazepam, alprazolam) and gamma-aminobutyric acid inhibitors (baclofen, tizanidine).

BIBLIOGRAPHY

1. Bell S, Kolobova I, Crapper L, Ernst C. Lesch-Nyhan syndrome: Models, theories, and therapies. Mol Syndromol. 2016;7(6):302-11.
2. Benz CM, Reeka-Bartschmid AM, Agostini FG. Case report: The Lesch-Nyhan syndrome. Eur J Paediatr Dent. 2004;5(2):110-14.
3. Neychev VK, Mitev VI. The biochemical basis of the neurobehavioral abnormalities in the Lesch-Nyhan syndrome: A hypothesis. Med Hypotheses. 2004;63(1):131-4.

Case 10.3

Nucleoside Analogues as Anticancer Drugs

COMPETENCY

- ❖ **BC10.1:** Describe nucleotides and nucleic acids and their clinical significance

Integration with Medicine

- ❖ **GM13.14:** Describe the indications for surgery, radiation and chemotherapy for common malignancies

Case Scenario

A 42-year-old male presents with complain of blood in stool for last 4 months. He also noticed that there in significant weight loss during this period. Colonoscopy revealed descending colon mass and biopsy revealed adenocarcinoma. Treatment was started with combination of nucleoside analogues.

QUESTIONS

Q.1. What are nucleoside analogues, explain with appropriate examples?

Q.2. What is mechanism of action of nucleoside analogue?

Q.3. Why there is a need of combination of chemotherapeutic drugs?

ANSWERS

A.1. Nucleoside analogue are one of the important drugs used widely as anticancer and antiviral drugs. Nucleoside analogues mimic endogenous nucleosides, exploiting cellular metabolism and becoming incorporated into both DNA and RNA. This property makes nucleoside analogues effective at inhibiting viral replication and stopping cancer cell proliferation.

A.2. Cytotoxic nucleoside analogues and nucleobases were among the first chemotherapeutic agents used against cancer. These agents behave as antimetabolites, compete with physiological nucleosides, and incorporate themselves in place of natural nucleobases resulting in inhibition of replication (cancer cell growth).

A.3. Resistance to nucleoside analogue is quite common when given in isolation by host cells, that is why combination therapy is advised.

BIBLIOGRAPHY

1. Galmarini CM, Mackey JR, Dumontet C. Nucleoside analogues and nucleobases in cancer treatment. Lancet Oncol. 2002;3(7):415-24.
2. Jordheim LP, Durantel D, Zoulim F, et al. Advances in the development of nucleoside and nucleotide analogues for cancer and viral diseases. Nat Rev Drug Discov. 2013;12: 447-64.

GIVE REASONS WHY

Q.1. Adenosine deaminase deficiency (ADA) may cause impaired immunity.

Ans. ADA is present in high quantity in lymphocytes both T and B lymphocytes. Deficiency of ADA causes accumulation of adenosine and deoxy-ATP, which inhibits the synthesis of other nucleotides take dCTP. So ADA deficiency manifest as reduced lymphocytes causes immune deficiency.

Q.2. Fluorouracil is an anticancer drug.

Ans. Fluorouracil competitively inhibits thymidylate synthase, which is required to convert uridine into thymidine.

dUMP → dTMP → DNA synthesis → replication of cells

Q.3. Why the reaction catalyzed by phosphoribosyl diphosphate (PRPP) synthetase is not a committed step in de novo-synthesis of purines?

Ans. Committed step is that step the product of which results in completion of the pathway. Here synthesis of PRPP is not surely result in completion of de novo-synthesis of purine as PRPP can be utilized in salvage pathway. The reaction which is catalyzed by phosphoribosyl amidotransferase is the committed step of de novo-synthesis.

Q.4. Modification of histones proteins are required for regulation of molecular process.

Ans. Various type of histone proteins modification are related with regulation of molecular processes like:

- Acetylation—activation of transcription
- Phosphorylation—condensation of chromosomes
- ADP—ribosylation—DNA repair
- Methylation—gene repression
- Ubiquitination—repression of transcription

Q.5. ORI and ORE are similar in function.

Ans. ORI—also known as Ori-C site, it the site of origin in procaryotes and recognized by a specific protein known as DnaA protein, while ORE—origin replication element is present in eukaryotes recognized by origin recognition complex (ORC) proteins. ORI is usually one in number, while ORE is multiple in number.

Q.6. Replisome is required for replication.

Ans. Replisome is a complex of enzymes and other factors required for DNA replication is known as replisome. It include—helicase, topoisomerase, DNA, DNB, primase SSB (single strand binding protein).

Q.7. Continuous cell division in cancer cells.

Ans. Cancer cells have sufficient activity of telomerase. This enzyme is required for replication of ends of DNA segment as there is no template for telomere [5' and 3']. Telomerase act as reverse transcriptase, it provides RNA template and which the 5' or 3' ends replicates. Usually with age the activity of telomerase decreases, but as rule in cancer cell continued presence of this enzyme makes them immortal.

Q.8. Coding strand also known as antitemplate strand.

Ans. During transcription of the DNA strand provides basis or template, which transcribes m-RNA, another strand of DNA is quite similar as newly synthesized m-RNA, so also known as coding strand (similar as newly coded strand) as it does not take part in transcription known as antitemplate/nontemplate strand.

Q.9. Histones protein are the dominating proteins of chromosomes.

Ans. Histone proteins are rich in lysine and arginine both amino acids are positively charged amino acid, they form strong ionic interaction with phosphate rich DNA molecules and provides it stability.

Q.10. In eukaryotes post-transcriptional modification occurs as 5' caping and 3' tailing.

Ans. In eucaryotes 5' copping occurs with 7-methyl guanosine triphosphate and tailing at 3′ end with 20–250 adenylic acid nucleotides. Purpose of both these processes is to prevent m-RNA from 5' and 3' exonuclease activity.

Q.11. RNA molecules can act as ribozymes.

Ans. Most of the enzymes are protein in nature but some of the RNA molecules can also act as a catalyst known as ribozymes for example:

a. Small nuclear RNAs (snRNAs) in spliceosomes, have catalytic activity and proteins (snurps) require to stabilize the structure of spliceosomes.
b. RNAse P and RNAse D for post-transcriptional modification of r-RNA and t-RNA.
c. 23 S r-RNA and 28S r-RNA has peptidyl transferase activity during translation in prokaryotes and eukaryotes respectively.

Q.12. Formation of Apo-β-48 is an example of post-transcriptional modification.

Ans. Apo β gene is transcribed to m-RNA which codes for Apo-β-100 (100 kD) in liver, but in intestinal cell, post-transcriptional modification known as m-RNA editing takes place for primary transcript. Once primary transcript synthesized, one enzyme cytidine deaminase, act on CAA codon codes for glutamic acid to UAA (stop stop) and end the process of translation at that site, results in formation of 49 kD protein formation known as Apo-β-48.

Q.13. RNA can synthesize DNA.

Ans. Enzyme reverse transcriptase, usually present in retrovirus, transposons and in some tumor cells, can use RNA as a template and synthesizes it's complementary DNA after formation of complete RNA-DNA hybrid. RNA stand is hydrolyzed by RNAse-H and the remaining single DNA strand act as template to form second strand of DNA and this is how double-stranded DNA is synthesized from single-stranded RNA.

Q.14. t-RNA acts as an adapter molecule.

Ans. m-RNA, nucleotide codon does not have affinity for amino acids, so amino acids for protein synthesis cannot directly bind to m-RNA. Then t-RNA act as an adapter or mediator between m-RNA and amino acids, it is through anticodon arm. Recognizes the codons on m-RNA and accordingly through its accepter arm from 3' OH end binds to amino acid and bring it to the m-RNA template for process of translation.

Q.15. A codon is a triplet sequence.

Ans. A codon, codes for an amino acids, 21 amino acids are present in a proteins. However, there is no codon for 21st amino acid selenocysteine, to code 20 amino acids, minimum 20 codons are needed. There are four different types of nucleotides present in DNA, which takes parts in codon formation. If, we assume that a pair of nucleotide can act as a codon, then, minimum possible combinations are $(4)^2 = 16$, which are less than existing amino acids. So, if move to 3 nucleotides then minimum possible combination will be $(4)^3 = 64$, that is how we can say that minimum number of nucleotides in a codon will be 3.

Q.16. Minimum 32 t-RNA are required to read the complete genetic code.

Ans. In the genetic code a total of 64 codons are present out of which three are stop stops and 61 are actual codons which need to be identified by t-RNA. To recognize these 61 codons, minimum 32t-RNAs are required this can be explained on the basis of wobble hypothesis.

Depending upon the nature of nucleotides at 5' end of anticodon, more than one codon can be recognized by a single t-RNA. So, if two codons are same at first two nucleotides and differ only at 3rd nucleotide (5′- 3′) can be identified by a single t-RNA.

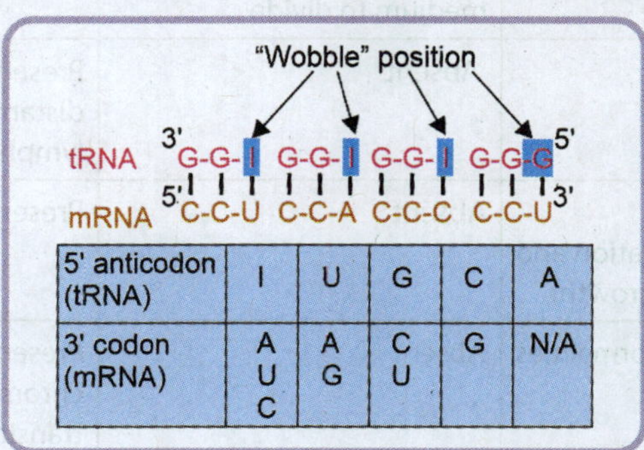

5' anticodon (tRNA)	I	U	G	C	A
3' codon (mRNA)	A U C	A G	C U	G	N/A

Q.17. Specific sequence on m-RNA is required to start the process of translation.

Ans. Two specific sequences are present on m-RNA to recognize initiation codon AUG. These are:

1. **Shine-Dalgarno sequence** in prokaryotes which is made from 4–9 purine basis and about 8 to13 base pair upstream (5') to the initiation codon AUG. This is recognized by 30 S r-RNA, which form a temporary base pairing with m-RNA through this sequence and stabilizes m-RNA between the cleft of 30 S and 50 S r-RNA.
2. **Kozak sequence in eukaryotes:** GCC A/G CC^{-1} $AUGG^{+4}$. AUG initiation codon is a part of Kozak sequence itself.

Q.18. Protein synthesis occurs through formation of polysomes.

Ans. One strand of m-RNA can be translated a number of times at the same time. It means a number of protein molecules can be synthesized from one strand of m-RNA at a particular time. Frequency to synthesize one protein molecule by one ribosome is 5–6 peptide bonds per second. Distance between two ribosomes on m-RNA remains about 80–100 nucleotides. Ribosomes attaches to the smooth endoplasmic reticulum.

During protein formation, functioning ribosome's moves over m-RNA till it reaches to stop codon. This movement of ribosome's exposes the initiation codon AUG so that the new ribosome complex can start the formation of second polypeptide/molecule of protein.

Q.19. Cancer cells are significantly different from normal cells.

Ans. Cancer cells show significant difference with normal cells. The differences are as follows:

S. No.	*Features*	*Normal cells*	*Cancer cell*
1.	Life span	Finite as their division depend upon mitogens (growth promoting factors)	Immortal as they need not mitogens for division
2.	Contact inhibition	Present growth of cells inhibited as they come in contact with other cells	Absent
3.	Anchorage dependence	Present need a solid medium to divide	Absent
4.	Metastasis	Absent	Present cancer cells can travel to distant tissues through blood or lymph
5.	Anaplasia (dedifferentiation and disordered growth)	Absent	Present
6.	Genetic abnormalities	Absent	Present such as abnormal chromosomal number deletion, translocation gene amplification or extrachromosomal genetic elements
7.	Biochemical changes		
	a. Rate of glycolysis, β-oxidation	Normal	Increased
	b. DNA and RNA content	Normal	Increased
	c. Abnormal proteins	Not present	Expressed

Q.20. Oncogene is an abnormal form of proto-oncogene.

Ans. Oncogene is produced by mutational activation of certain genes, known as proto-oncogenes. This can be done by:

a. Point mutation
b. Gene amplification
c. Gene rearrangements
d. Insertion of viral promoter

Q.21. P53 gene is known as guardian of genome.

Ans. Mutation in p53 gene can result in wide range of tumors. Change in the sequence of this gene is the most common cause for spontaneous cancers. The product of this gene is a cell cycle regulator protein, required to check the damage in DNA before replication. It is a check point between G1 and S phase of the cell cycle. If any damage in DNA sequence is detected, the product protein arrests the G1 phase so that sufficient time can be available to correct the damage or it may stimulate the process of apoptosis (programmed cell death).

Q.22. Inclusion cell disease is the result due to defect in protein targeting.

Ans. Absence of signal peptide in newly synthesized proteins, makes them unable to reach their target area of function and result in various diseases.

Defect in protein targeting may cause:

1. Inclusion cell disease—mannose-6-phosphatase not being able to reach lysosomes.
2. Zellweger syndrome—absence of enzymes in peroxisomes required to metabolized long chain fatty acids
3. Primary hyperoxaluria—enzyme alanine glyoxylate aminotransferase present in mitochondria instead of peroxisomes.

Q.23. Antibiotics as prescribed dose is usually nontoxic to human being.

Ans. Most of the antibiotics act by inhibiting protein synthesis, they act on 70 S ribosomes and not on 80 S ribosomes (present in eukaryotes).

Antibiotics

Bacteriostatic:

Tetracyclines—inhibit 30 S subunit of bacterial ribosome and inhibit attachment of amino acyl t-RNA to A site.

Chloramphenicol—inhibit peptidyl transferase of bacterial ribosome.

Erythromycin and clindamycin—prevent translocation process.

Bactericidal:

Streptomycin and aminoglycoside—binds with 30 S subunit and cause misreading of m-RNA.

However, there are some inhibitors of protein synthesis in eukaryotes which are usually not of clinical use, e.g., Puromycin—premature separation of peptide chain as it is structurally similar as tyrosine t-RNA. Cycloheximide—inhibit peptidyl transferase.

Q.24. Proteome of an organism depends upon genome.

Ans. Total genetic information present in a cell is known as genome, while total of expressed proteins in a cell is known as proteome. Proteins expression depends upon genome, however unlike genome, which is same in all cells of the organism, proteome (expression of protein) is different in different cells, depending upon the regulators of gene expression.

Q.25. Synthetic antisense nucleic acid strands are used as a therapeutic tool.

Ans. To manipulate the expression of certain genes, e.g., in HIV or cancer (small strand) oligonucleotide strand of DNA or RNA is used, which is also known as synthetic antisense nucleic acid strand. These single stranded oligonucleotides bind with m-RNA transcribed from a particular gene and trap its function to synthesize protein.

Q.26. Vectors used for recombinant DNA technology have some essential properties.

Ans. Cloning vectors for the recombinant DNA technology may be plasmid, bacteriophage or a cosmid. The following essential properties are present in a vector:

a. At least one specific palindromic region
b. Capable of autonomous replication
c. A specific property like antibiotic resistance which could be used to find the presence of inserted foreign DNA

Q.27. Why child is not exactly like a parents?

Ans. During gamete formation or during meiosis, exchange of genetic information occurs through crossover, between two homologous chromosomes. Such recombination of specific loci of two homologous chromosomes, explains child is not exactly like parents.

Q.28. Retinoblastoma (RB) protein prevents cancer.

Ans. RB protein is a product of onco-suppressor gene. It regulates cell cycle. It binds with transcription factor E2F and makes it inactive and inhibits G_1 phase of cell cycle. In a regular/controlled cycle cyclin-D levels in later stage of G_1 inactivates RB protein and allow cell cycle to move normally. After certain viral infection (SV40, HSV, HPV), the viral protein may combine with RB protein and make it unable to inhibit cell cycle at G_1 phase and results in cancer.

Q.29. Enzymes used in recombination DNA technology is known as restriction endonuclease.

Ans. Enzymes used in this technique are also known as molecular scissors as they cut the DNA fragment from specific site which is a palindromic sequence and insert or add that segment into vectors for further multiplication. As these enzymes obtained from bacteria and restrict the entry of phages into bacterial cell and prevent the viral or bacteriophage multiplication into bacterial cells itself, they are known as restriction endonuclease.

Q.30. Insertional inactivation of certain gene use as marker for hybrid DNA.

Ans. During the process of DNA recombination gene of interest is obtained from DNA segment and is inserted into vectors (plasmids, bacteriophages or cosmids), at their specific site where they inactivate the particular gene known as insertional inactivation. This is further used to identify which host cell get transfected with required vectors, e.g., a plasmid pBR325 vector has Apr (ampicillin resistance), Tcr (Tetracycline resistance), CmR (chloramphenicol resistance).

The restriction endonuclease EcoRI inserts the gene of interest in the CmR, so vector loses this property of chloramphenicol resistance. Once these hybrid/chimeric plasmids enter into *E. coli* through transfection, to find out which colony of *E. coli* contain hybrid plasmid CmR resistance is used to differentiate these colonies from other.

Q.31. Stem cells shows developmental plasticity.

Ans. Stem cells have specific property of renewal (capacity to produce unaltered daughter cells) as well as to generate variety of specialized cells under the influence of specific stimulus this second property is known as developmental plasticity.

- **Totipotent:** Capable of producing all type of cells
- **Pluripotent:** Capable to generate cells of three germ cells
- **Multipotent:** Capable to produce closely related cells
- **Unipotent:** Capable to produce one type of cell

Q.32. DNA fingerprinting is also known as DNA profile.

Ans. In every individual, short and repeated sequences of nucleotide present which is scattered in various sites. These are known as Tandem repeats. These repeats are unique for an individual, also known DNA profile of an individual. It is used to find culprit of crime, to solve dispute of parenthood.

Q.33. Polymorphism and mutation are not same.

Ans. Any alteration in a gene sequence if occurs in more than 1% of population and usually not fetal, is known as polymorphism, while if this change occur in an individual with deleterious effect is known as mutation.

Q.34. DNA polymerase III is the predominant enzyme of replication in prokaryotes.

Ans. DNA polymerase III has

a. 3' to 5' ex-nuclease activity that is needed for proofreading of the process.
b. Rate of replication is maximum-600-1,000 nucleotides/second.
c. Processivity is maximum—that is dissociation of enzyme after addition of how many nucleotides in newly synthesized DNA segment. It is about 5,00,000 nucleotides.

Q.35. DNA polymerase I is the dominating enzyme for DNA ligation, along with DNA ligase.

Ans. DNA ligation is needed for lagging strand where DNA is replicated in fragments known as Okazaki segments. DNA polymerase I through it's 5'- 3' exonuclease activity removes primers of each Okazaki fragment, replicate the gap generated through its polymerase activity. Finally, the nick between two segments is sealed with DNA ligase.

Q.36. Lack of telomerase activity may contribute in cell aging.

Ans. The terminal ends of chromosomes are known as telomere, which is characterized as 500 to 5,000 times repeated sequence of $(TTAGGG)_n$ at 5' end and its complimentary sequence at 3' end. DNA polymerase does not replicate these terminal sequences. Specific enzyme telomerase is required to replicate these sequences as this enzyme has an integral sequence of RNA template, that is used to synthesize the ends. So, we can say that telomerase acts as reverse transcriptase and required to maintain the length of chromosomes during replication. Decrease activity of telomerase results in shortening/short-length of chromosome in each replication and causes cell aging.

Q.37. There is no codon for selenocysteine.

Ans. Selenocysteine is 21st amino acid, however there is no specific codon for this. It is found on active sites of following enzymes: (1) Thioredoxin reductase, (2) Glutathione peroxidase, (3) Deiodinase and (4) Selenoprotein P, a glycoprotein seen in mammalian blood.

As there is no specific codon. Selenocysteine is synthesized as co-translational modification. Under the influence of specific stimulus stop codon UGA, gives signal to tRNA to carry selenocysteine (selenium containing), instead of serine. It means the tRNA which normally transfer serine to m-RNA. Now this t-RNA will carry selenocysteine to m-RNA and how this serine gets converted into selenocysteine.

Se + ATP ⟶ Se – p + AMP + Pi (selenium gets activated)

Serine + Se – p ⟶ Selenocysteine + pi (oxygen atom of –OH group of serine is replaced with "se")

Q.38. Mushroom poisoning is lethal.

Ans. Alpha amanitin, a toxin from mushroom inactivates RNA polymerase-II. And inhibit the process of transcription and further the protein synthesis.

Q.39. Cancer are multifactorial in origin.

Ans. Cancer can be due to:

a. Mutagens—substances which can increase the rate of mutations, e.g., X-rays, ϒ-rays, dyes, toxins, food additives, etc.
b. Oncogenic virus:
   1. Epstein–Barr virus Burkitt's lymphoma, nasopharyngeal carcinoma
   2. HPV—human papilloma virus-uterine, cervical carcinoma
   3. HBV—hepatitis B virus—hepatoma
c. Oncogenes—genes capable of causing cancer. Most of the genes are present as proto-oncogenes, which after getting stimulus get converted into oncogenes.
d. Onco-suppressor genes—these genes normally protect the cancer but once deleted, mutated, they results in cancer.

Q.40. Genome, genomic and genetics are not same.

Ans. Total DNA present in a cell including nucleus and mitochondria is known as genome. Study of this genome is known as genomics, examining the sequence and function of a single gene is known as genetics.

Gene therapy is an advancement in DNA recombinant DNA technology.

Section 11

Miscellaneous

- **Case 11.1:** Bacterial Meningitis
- **Case 11.2:** Chronic Renal Failure
- **Case 11.3:** Nephrotic Syndrome

Give Reasons Why

Case 11.1

Bacterial Meningitis

COMPETENCY

- **BC14.17:** Describe briefly various body fluids and discuss the composition of CSF

Integration with Medicine

- **GM4.6** Discuss the approach to the patient with Acute Febrile Illness
- **GM17.7** Enumerate the indication of lumbar puncture and describe the findings in CSF in different types of meningitis
- **GM26.12** Describe and discuss the common causes, clinical features and management of encephalitis and meningitis

Case Scenario

A 24-year-old female presents to the emergency department with complains of high grade fever with chills, worsening headache, neck pain, and back pain of 2 days duration. In addition, she reports 3 to 4 episodes of nausea and vomiting and difficulty maintaining her balance. on examination there is swallowing over right eye and neck rigidity is present.

In addition to blood and urine investigation, lumber puncture was done, and CSF is send for analysis.

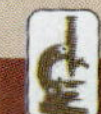

Laboratory Findings Reveal

Blood examination

- Complete blood count—13,000 cells/cumm (5,000–11,000 cells/cumm)
- Differential count shows increased neutrophils
- ESR—70 mm/1st hr (1–20 mm/1st hr)

Urine examination

- Urine sugar—negative
- Urine protein—negative
- Pus cell—1–2 cells/hpf
- RBC—NIL

CSF analysis

- CSF total count—20 cell/cumm (0–8 cell/cumm)
- CSF glucose—32 mg/dL (40–80 mg/dL)
- CSF protein—52 mg/dL (10–40 mg/dL)

QUESTIONS

Q.1. What is the most probable diagnosis?

Q.2. What are the causes and risk factors of above clinical condition?

Q.3. What are the other investigations required in such a clinical case?

Q.4. What is the line of management of such patients?

ANSWERS

A.1. Patients is most probably suffering from bacterial meningitis. Meningitis is defined as inflammation of the meninges. The meninges are the three membranes (the dura mater, arachnoid mater, and piamater) that line the vertebral canal and skull enclosing the brain and spinal cord. Encephalitis, on the other hand, is inflammation of the brain itself. Clinical presentation of bacterial meningitis is summarized in **Figure 11.1.1.**

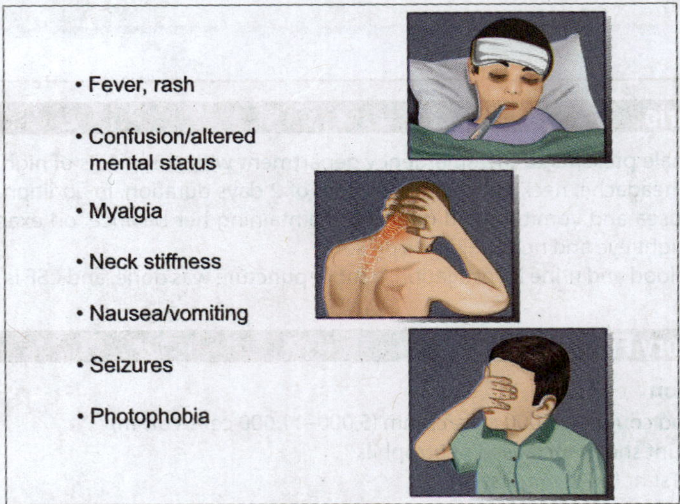

Fig. 11.1.1: Clinical presentation of bacterial meningitis.

A.2. Meningitis can be caused by infectious and noninfectious processes (autoimmune disorders, cancer/paraneoplastic syndromes, drug reactions). Infectious agents of meningitis include bacteria, viruses, fungi, and less commonly parasites.

Risk factors for meningitis include:

- Chronic medical disorders (renal failure, diabetes, adrenal insufficiency, cystic fibrosis)
- Extremes of age
- Immunosuppressed states (iatrogenic, transplant recipients, congenital immunodeficiencies, AIDS)

- Bacterial endocarditis
- Malignancy
- IV drug use
- Sickle cell anemia
- Splenectomy

A.3. Meningitis is diagnosed through CSF analysis. The CSF findings expected in bacterial, viral, and fungal meningitis are shown in **Table 11.1.1**.

Table 11.1.1: CSF finding in bacterial, viral, fungal meningitis.

	Appearance	*Opening pressure (mm Hg)*	*WBC (cell/mL)*	*Protein (mg/dL)*	*Glucose (mg/dL)*
Normal	Clear	90–180	<8	15–45	50–80
Bacterial meningitis	Turbid	Elevated	>1,000–2,000	>200	<40
Viral meningitis	Clear	Normal	<300; lymphocytic predominance	<200	Normal
Fungal meningitis	Clear	Normal-elevated	<500	>200	Normal-low

A.4. Mainstay of the management of meningitis is antibiotics and supportive care, in addition fever control, IV fluids and symptomatic care is essential in case of meningitis.

BIBLIOGRAPHY

1. Hersi K, Gonzalez FJ, Kondamudi NP. Meningitis. [Updated 2022 Aug 14]. In: StatPearls [Internet]. Treasure Island (FL): StatPearls Publishing; 2022. Available from: https://www.ncbi.nlm.nih.gov/books/NBK459360/
2. Hoffman O, Weber RJ. Pathophysiology and treatment of bacterial meningitis. Ther Adv Neurol Disord. 2009;2(6):1-7.

Case 11.2

Chronic Renal Failure

COMPETENCY

- ❖ **BC11.1:** Describe the function tests of kidney, liver, thyroid and adrenal glands and their clinical significance. Interpret the function tests report
- ❖ **BC14.19:** Explain the basis and rationale of biochemical tests done and interpretation of laboratory results in Renal failure

Integration with Medicine

- ❖ **GM10.5:** Describe and discuss the pathophysiology and clinical findings of uraemia

Case Scenario

A 60-year-old female admitted in the hospital with chief complaints of shortness of breath, confusion, and fever since last 3 days. She had a past history of hypertension and diabetes of 7 years for which she is on medication. On examination facial puffiness and pedal edema present.

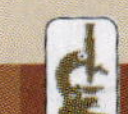

Laboratory Findings Reveal

- Serum creatinine—6.9 mg/dL (0.4–1.2 mg/dL)
- Blood urea—149 mg/dL (10–40 mg/dL)
- Serum calcium—6.8 mg/dL (9–11 mg/dL)
- Na^+—139 mEq/L (136–145 mEq/L)
- K^+—5.4 mEq/L (3.5–5 mEq/L)
- Urinary protein—present
- Estimated GFR—64 mL/min

QUESTIONS

Q.1. What is the probable diagnosis? Enumerate the causes of such clinical condition.

Q.2. How the disease can be assessed?

Q.3. What is the line of management for this patient?

ANSWERS

A.1. Probable diagnosis is chronic renal disease. There is a significant irreversible reduction in number and function of nephrons.

Causes of CKD may be:

- Diabetes mellitus
- Hypertension
- Primary glomerulonephritis
- Chronic tubulointerstitial nephritis
- Hereditary or cystic diseases
- Secondary glomerulonephritis or vasculitis
- Plasma cell dyscrasias or neoplasm
- Sickle cell nephropathy (SCN)

Early deterioration of renal function due to primary causes, secondary progressive mechanism takes place which causes hypertrophy of remaining nephrons to compensate for the loss, but in later stages of disease, this fails lead to renal failure. Clinical presentation of CRF is summarized in **Table 11.2.1**.

Table 11.2.1: Clinical presentation of chronic kidney disease.

• Nausea • Vomiting • Loss of appetite • Fatigue and weakness • Sleep disturbance • Oliguria • Decreased mental sharpness • Muscle twitches and cramps • Swelling of feet and ankles • Persistent pruritus • Chest pain due to uremic pericarditis	• Shortness of breath due to pulmonary edema from fluid overload • Hypertension that's difficult to control • Skin pigmentation • Scratch marks from pruritus • Pericardial friction rub due to uremic pericarditis • Uremic frost, where high levels of BUN result in urea in sweat • Hypertensive fundal changes suggesting chronicity

A.2. CKD can be assessed by **(Table 11.2.2)**:

a. **Proteinuria:** Microalbuminuria is an early indicator for renal disease. Excretion of 30–300 mg of albumin/day is known as microalbuminuria. In later stages of renal disease there may be mild to massive proteinuria.

b. **GFR:** Glomerular filtration rate—is the rate in mL/min that substances are cleared from circulation by kidney glomeruli.

Glomerular filtration rate (GFR) ≈ 125 mL/min

Table 11.2.2: Classification of chronic kidney disease based on glomerular filtration rate.

Stages	*GFR mL/min*
1	>/90
2	60–89
3	30–59
4	15–29
5	<15

Source: NKF KDOQI guidelines.

c. **Protein/creatinine** (albumin mg/creatinine g) ratio >68—males and >107-females indicate significant renal damage normal ratio 15-68 mg/g and 10-107 mg/g in males and females respectively.

A.3. Management of CKD principally depends on its etiology. Most often management consists of measures to help control signs and symptoms, reduce complications, and slow progression of the disease.

1. Treatment of underlying causes (hypertension, cardiovascular disease, diabetes mellitus)
2. Treatment of complications (anemia, edema, bone, and mineral disorder)
3. Dietary management—restriction of protein diet to minimize waste, minimize phosphate and aluminum containing phosphate binding antaacids. Adequate calcium (1-2 g/day) and calcitriol intake (0.25-1.0 μg/day).
4. Treatment of end-stage renal failure (dialysis, kidney transplant).

BIBLIOGRAPHY

1. Vaidya SR, Aeddula NR. Chronic renal failure. [Updated 2022 Aug 10]. In: StatPearls [Internet]. Treasure Island (FL): StatPearls Publishing; 2022. Available from: https://www.ncbi.nlm.nih.gov/books/NBK535404/
2. Webster AC, Nagler EV, Morton RL, Masson P. Chronic kidney disease. Lancet. 2017;389(10075):1238-52.

Case 11.3

Nephrotic Syndrome

COMPETENCY

❖ **BC14.19:** Explain the basis and rationale of biochemical tests done and interpretation of laboratory results in Nephrotic syndrome

Integration with Medicine

❖ **GM10.1:** Define, describe, classify, differentiate between the pathophysiologic causes of acute and chronic renal failure

Case Scenario

A 5-year-old male with weight of 20 kg brought to medicine OPD with complains of swelling over face and pitting edema was present over lower limbs. Parents revealed the history of oliguria in the last few days.

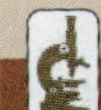

Laboratory Findings Reveal

- Total protein—3.5 g/dL (6–8 g/dL)
- Serum albumin—2 g/dL (3.5–5 g/dL)
- Total cholesterol—342 mg/dL (<200 mg/dL)
- LDL cholesterol—196 mg/dL (<100 mg/dL)
- Triglycerides—329 mg/dL (<150 mg/dL)
- Urinary glucose—Nil
- Urinary protein—+++

QUESTIONS

Q.1. What is the probable diagnosis? Explain the biochemical basis.

Q.2. Explain the basis of proteinuria and abnormal lipid profile in this patient.

Q.3. What treatment should be advised to the patients?

ANSWERS

A.1. The probable diagnosis is nephrotic syndrome. Nephrotic syndrome is usually a chronic condition that eventually lead to chronic progressive renal failure.

Causes of Nephrotic Syndrome

Primary nephrotic syndrome is idiopathic.

Chronic glomerulopathies, damage to glomerulus by toxin and drugs, immune complex mediated, diabetic nephropathy can lead to nephrotic syndrome.

In children, it may result after a viral infection (high grade fever with chills and rigors) or with preceding allergy. This may cause cytokine related immune injury to the glomerulus membrane. Which further results in alteration in the charge of protein molecules as well as the podocyte integrity, this may cause increase permeability of glomerulus membrane **(Fig. 11.3.1)**.

- Edema (around eyes, ankle and feet)
- Proteinuria
- Hypoalbuminemia
- Hyperlipidemia
- Hypercoagulable state (loss of clotting factor)
- Arterial and venous thromboembolism
- Increased risk of bacterial infection
- Renal failure

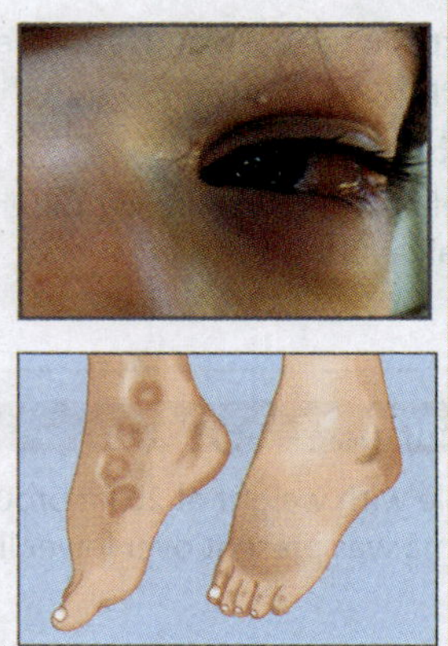

Fig. 11.3.1: Clinical presentation of nephrotic syndrome.

A.2. In healthy person proteins are not excreted out in urine. Two important factors that prevent the filtration of serum proteins through glomerulus membrane:

a. Large size of proteins (albumin is smallest and that is the reason it comes out in urine earliest in renal disease).

b. Charge over the protein particles that causes repulsion from the proteins of glomerular membrane.

But in case of certain conditions, glomerulitis (infection), nephrotic syndrome (infection or preceding allergy), there may be increase in pore size of glomerulus and in diabetic nephropathy (glycation of glomerulus protein) there is reduction in repulsion between protein molecules. This further causes excretion of proteins in urine.

Excess excretion of proteins in urine causes a decrease in osmotic pressure and viscosity of blood which may be a stimulus for increase hepatic lipogenesis. The other causes may be loss of lipo regulatory substances in urine. Both these two factors result in increased level of lipid parameters in blood.

A.3. Management of primary glomerular disease consists of supportive management and disease modifying specific therapy.

Supportive Therapy

Supportive therapy is aimed at controlling blood pressure, relieving edema, reduction of proteinuria and hyperlipidemia, and management of any other metabolic derangement that may be present.

Specific Therapy

1. Steroid therapy
2. Immunosuppressive drugs
3. Inhibitors of renin-angiotensin system
4. Anticoagulants for hypercoagulable state, if required.

For secondary glomerular disease, the focus is to aggressively manage the underlying causes such as underlying infection.

BIBLIOGRAPHY

1. Khanna R. Clinical presentation and management of glomerular diseases: Hematuria, nephritic and nephrotic syndrome. Mo Med. 2011;108(1):33-6.
2. Orth SR, Ritz E. The nephrotic syndrome. N Engl J Med. 1998;338:1202.

GIVE REASONS WHY

Q.1. Anemia is seen in chronic renal failure (CRF).

Ans. This may be due to deficiency of erythropoietin a protein synthesized from renal parenchymal cells. In chronic renal failure, there may be defects in synthesis of erythropoietin. This protein is further required from proliferation and differentiation of erythroid precursors, regulate the process of erythropoiesis, number of RBC in peripheral blood. That's why its deficiency leads to anemia.

ENVIRONMENTAL POLLUTION

Q.1. Anemia occurs in lead poisoning.

Ans. Lead inhibits heme synthesis. It is an inhibitor aminolevulinic acid synthase and ALA dehydratase, also the enzyme ferro chelatase. Decrease heme synthesis causes anemia. There is no safe limit of lead levels in blood. Levels up to 10 mg/dL is tolerable, more than that is toxic. Besides anemia it may results in neurological manifestation as well as mental retardation in children.

Q.2. Minamata disease is due to poisoning with organic mercury.

Ans. Organic mercury in the form of fungicides, industrial waste, excreted into sea. This enters into fish and eating such fish causes poisoning with organic mercury. It is commonly seen in the population living around Minamata Bay, that is why known as Minamata disease. The classical signs of disease are dysarthria, ataxia and visual field defect. Normal levels of mercury is less than 1 mg/dL >2–5 mg/dL is toxic, 15 mg/dL or more that that is fatal.

Q.3. Consumption of raw cabbage causes goiter formation.

Ans. High consumption of goitrogenic foods such as cabbage, maize, sweet potato, and millet. The goitrogenic foods contain thiocyanate and isothiocyanate that restrain thyroid iodide transport. This will results into thyroid hormone deficiency and goiter.

Q.4. Consumption of Khesari dal may cause paralysis of lower limbs.

Ans. Khesari dal also known as *Lathyrus sativus*. It contains a neurotoxin (beta oxalyl amino alanine). This can be separated from dal through cooking or decanting the supernatant. This toxic inhibits lysyl oxidase, reduces cross linking in collagen, also having neurotoxicity and cause damage of upper motor neurons, result in paralysis of lower limbs.

Q.5. Serum screening should be done in high-risk pregnancy.

Ans. To rule out any chromosomal abnormality five analytes need to be estimated in maternal blood along with USG in case of high-risk pregnancy:

(1) Alpha fetoprotein (AFP), (2) human chorionic gonadotropin (Beta-hCG), (3) unconjugated estriol (uE3), (4) inhibin and (5) pregnancy associated plasma protein (PAPP).

NUTRITION

Q.1. The values of specific dynamic action (SDA) are maximum for proteins.

Ans. SDA is the production of heat following the intake of food. This is about 30% for proteins, 15% for lipids, and 5% for carbohydrates. Proteins being a complex molecule energy require for its digestion, absorption, and transport in more than other biomolecules.

Q.2. Mutual supplementation of some proteins is advised.

Ans. Some proteins are deficient in certain amino acids and can limit the growth of a person, such amino acids are known as limiting amino acids. To over cum this problem a mixture of proteins is advised to gain the proper growth, e.g.,

Protein with limiting amino acids		*Proteins need to be supplemented in*
Rice	Lysine, threonine	Pulse
Wheat	Lysine, threonine	Pulse
Pulse (Bengal)	Cysteine, methionine	Cereals

Q.3. Glycemic index is lower for complex blood.

Ans. Glycemic index is a ratio of:

$$\frac{\text{Increase in blood glucose level after taking test meal (50 g)}}{\text{Increase in blood glucose after taking glucose meal (50 g)}}$$

If we take complex food the increase in blood glucose will be less as it takes time for the food to be digested and absorbed through the intestine.

Q.4. Total energy requirement of an individual is not only dependent on basal metabolic rate (BMR).

Ans. BMR is energy required to sustain the vital functions of the body [such as pumping of heart, gastrointestinal (GI) motility, breathing, and conduction of nerve impulse] during complete physical and mental rest. However, besides BMR, an individual need energy expended as SDA (specific dynamic action—energy used in digestion, absorption, transport, and storage of food biomolecules) as well as energy required for physical activity.

Energy requirement during moderate physical work of a 70 kg body weight person.

1. BMR ≈ 1,680 kcal/24 hrs.
2. Physical activity (40% of BMR) ≈ 670 kcal.
3. SDA (10% BMR) ≈ 235 kcal

Total ≈ 2,585 kcal

Q.5. Net protein utilization (NPU) is a better index than biologic value (BV) for the assessment of protein quality.

Ans. $\text{Biologic value} = \frac{\text{Nitrogen retained}}{\text{Nitrogen absorbed}} \times 100$

$$\text{Net protein} = \frac{\text{Nitrogen retained}}{\text{Nitrogen ingested}} \times 100$$

NPU also indicates the amount of nitrogen lost during digestion.

Q.6. Why there is inflammation and arthritis occurs in gout?

Ans. Urate crystals are deposited in synovial fluid. These are phagocytosed by inflammatory cells and cause physical damage to lysosomes in these cells. This result in release of enzymes from lysosomes causes inflammation and arthritis.

Q.7. Cathepsins are implicated in tumor metastasis.

Ans. Cathepsins are the most abundant lysosomal proteases that are mainly found in acidic endo/lysosomal compartments where they play a vital role in intracellular protein degradation. Cathepsins are proteolytically active when attached to other cell surface proteins. This extracellular activity allows cancer cells to invade surrounding tissues, blood, and lymph vessels and metastasize to distant sites.

Q.8. Decreased lung elasticity in silicosis.

Ans. Silica is a substance naturally found in certain types of stone, rock, sand and clay. Working with these materials can create a very fine dust that can be easily inhaled. Once inside the lungs, it causes swelling (inflammation) and gradually leads to areas of hardened and scarred lung tissue (fibrosis) also known as silicosis.

Q.9. Animals of polar region can maintain their body temperature.

Ans. Animals of polar regain have brown adipose tissue which contain an uncoupling protein (UCPS) known as thermogenin, which uncouples the process of ETC and phosphorylation by forming an alternate proton channel in the inner mitochondrial membrane. So, the protons instead of passing through ATP synthase, moves from this channel and there will be no ATP formation takes place and energy releases as heat. Uncouplers just uncouple ETC with phosphorylation. It means ETC goes on as such as it is not coupled with ATP formation (phosphorylation), the energy will not trap as ATP and releases as heat energy.

Other examples of uncouplers are:

a. DNA (Dinitrophenol), DNC (Dinitro cresol)—increases the permeability of IMM for protons, inhibits generation of protein gradient.
b. Physiological uncoupler—free fatty acids, bilirubin and thyronine.
c. Ionophore-gramicidin and valinomycin—they dissipate the proton gradient and prevent ATP synthesis.

Q.10. Mitochondrial DNA is about 10 times susceptible to mutations than nuclear DNA.

Ans. Electron transport chain takes place in mitochondria it's DNA is at high risk for the exposure of free radicals and oxygen reactive species that's why chances of mutation is mare in mitochondrial DNA. This is also known as mitochondrial myopathies.

Q.11. Amount of ATP made from NADH+H$^+$ is more than $FADH_2$.

Ans. NADH + H$^+$ enters in ETC through complex I , while $FADH_2$ enters through complex II.

Protons pumps through complexes are as follows.

Complexes	*Number of protons pump*
I	**4**
II	**NIL**
III	**2**
IV	**4**

So total protons pumped into inter mitochondrial space are 10 and 6 when NADH + H$^+$ and $FADH_2$ enters in ETC, respectively. When these protons re-enter in mitochondrial matrix through ATP synthetase ,10 protons generate 2.5 ATPs and 6 protons generate 1.5 ATPs.

Q.12. Cyanide is a deadly poison.

Ans. Cyanide is the permanent inhibitor of complex IV of ETC. that is how it inhibits the electron flow and then the ATP formation. Besides cyanide, there are some other inhibitors of ETC complexes:

Complex I—Rotenone (a fish poison), Barbiturates, BAL (British anti-Lewisite)

Complex II—Melonate

Complex III—Antimycin

Complex IV—H_2S, carbon monoxide

Q.13. Duchenne muscular dystrophy mainly affects boys in early age.

Ans. Duchenne muscular dystrophy is X-linked recessive disease. So females are usually acted as carrier while males are affected with disease. This is characterized by mutation in a gene code for dystrophin protein. This protein maintains the connection of cytoskeleton of cells which it's basal lamina of extracellular matrix. The abnormal form of protein causes excess calcium to enter into the cell, which may further lead to water intake into mitochondria and destruction of mitochondria.

Q.14. Copper irons are required for maturation of collagen.

Ans. Collagen is synthesized in the cell in pre-procollagen form. Post-translation modification occurs in the form of hydroxylation of lysine and proline residues. Vitamin C, iron and copper are essential for these modifications.

Q.15. Osteogenesis imperfecta is a collagen disorder.

Ans. There is a genetic defect (mutation in DNA) replaces glycine with cysteine in type I collagen. This may cause partial unfolding of the polypeptides in collagen, results in defective collagen. As collagen type I present in bones it causes fragile and brittle bones with multiple fractures known as osteogenesis imperfecta.

Q.16. Inulin is an ideal marker to measure urinary clearance and glomerular filtration rate.

Ans. Inulin is a homopolymer of fructose. It has all the characteristics of an ideal marker to measure urinary clearance.

- It cannot be metabolized in body
- Freely filtered from glomerular membrane
- Neither secreted not reabsorbed by renal tubular epithelial cells.

Q.17. Why mannitol is given in treatment of subdural hemorrhage?

Ans. Mannitol may reduce subarachnoid space pressure by creating an osmotic gradient between the cerebrospinal fluid in the arachnoid space and the plasma.

Q.18. ORS is used in treatment of diarrhea causing dehydration.

Ans. ORS contain NaCl, KCl, Trisodium citrate and glucose. NaCl and KCl maintain the electrolyte balance, trisodium citrate increase shelf-life of ORS. The combination optimizes the absorption of fluid in the intestines, which helps quickly replenish fluids.

Q.19. GAGs (Glycosaminoglycans) acts as lubricant.

Ans. GAGs contain large number of negatively charged groups (sulphate, carbonyl, acetylated, amino groups) in their structure and have tendency to absorb water molecules and so they produce viscous solution.

Q.20. Sucrose is an invert sugar.

Ans. Sucrose is dextrorotatory (+66.5o). Sucrose is hydrolyzed into glucose (+52.5o) and fructose (-92o), the levorotary effect of fructose is greater than dextrorotatory effect of glucose. So after hydrolysis sucrose in the solutions becomes levorotary, that is why it is known as Invert sugar.

Q.21. Sodium fluoride vial is used for estimation of glucose.

Ans. Sodium fluoride vial contain fluoride ions, which are inhibitors of glycolytic enzyme enolase. Thus through stopping glycolysis in red blood cells, it maintains the glucose level in the serum sample.

Q.22. Arachidonic acid is a semi-essential fatty acid.

Ans. Nutritionally essential fatty acids are linoleic acid and linolenic acid. These fatty acids cannot be synthesized in our body and has to be taken through diet. Arachidonic acid can be synthesized from linolenic acid but not in sufficient amount so again it also has to be supplemented in diet and known as semi-essential fatty acid.

Q.23. Keeping the fried namkeen for a longer duration in unvacuumed environment causes unpleasant taste and smell.

Ans. This is due to oxidative rancidity. Unsaturated fatty acids present in the food undergoes partial oxidation by environment air to form epoxides and peroxides as free radicals. Their formation may cause unpleasant smell and taste.

Q.24. Cardiolipin deficiency lead to heart failure.

Ans. Cardiolipin is a phospholipid also known as diphosphatidyl glycerol. It is rich in mitochondrial membrane of heart muscles. Deficiency of cardiolipin causes mitochondrial dysfunction and results in heart failure.

Index

Page numbers followed by *f* refer to figure, *fc* refer to flowchart, and *t* refer to table.

I